INTRODUCTION

Stroke, a severe and potentially life-altering medical event, occurs when blood flow to the brain is disrupted, either by a blockage in the blood vessels (ischemic stroke) or by bleeding within the brain (hemorrhagic stroke). A stroke can lead to a range of physical and cognitive impairments, making it crucial to adopt preventive measures and lifestyle changes to mitigate its risk. One integral component of stroke prevention and recovery is a well-considered stroke diet. Understanding the significance of a stroke diet requires acknowledging the intricate relationship between dietary choices and cardiovascular health. The brain, highly dependent on a steady blood supply, is vulnerable to the same risk factors that affect the heart and blood vessels. Consequently, dietary habits play a pivotal role in either promoting or undermining vascular health.

The primary goals of a stroke diet are twofold: first, to minimize the risk factors associated with stroke, and second, to support the recovery process in individuals who have experienced a stroke. A well-crafted stroke diet is about what to include and what to limit or avoid. It encompasses a balanced, heart-healthy approach, emphasizing nutrient-dense foods that contribute to overall well-being.

In this comprehensive exploration of the stroke diet, we will explore the fundamental principles guiding dietary choices for stroke prevention and recovery. From the incorporation of antioxidant-rich fruits and vegetables to the mindful selection of fats and proteins, each aspect of the stroke diet is intricately connected to the broader objective of safeguarding brain health. Moreover, we will explore the nuances of portion control, hydration, and the importance of consulting healthcare professionals for personalized dietary guidance.

Recognizing that stroke prevention and recovery extend beyond dietary considerations, this exploration will underscore the synergy between a stroke-conscious diet and other lifestyle factors. Regular physical activity, maintaining a healthy weight, and managing stress are integral components of a holistic approach to stroke care.

Embarking on a journey to understand the intricacies of the stroke diet is a step towards minimizing the risk of stroke and a commitment to fostering a lifestyle that nurtures the health and vitality of the entire cardiovascular system. As we navigate through the nuances of stroke prevention and recovery through dietary choices, we gain insights into a proactive and empowering approach to overall well-being.

CHAPTER ONE

What Is Stroke?

A stroke, often referred to as a "brain attack," is a critical and potentially debilitating medical event that unfolds in the intricate circuitry of the human brain. Characterized by a sudden disruption of blood flow to the brain, strokes manifest in two primary forms: ischemic and hemorrhagic.

TYPES OF STROKES

Strokes, often deemed as medical emergencies of paramount significance, come in distinct forms, each with its unique characteristics and implications. Understanding the types of strokes, primarily ischemic and hemorrhagic, is pivotal for effective management, prevention, and post-event care.

1. Ischemic Stroke:

• Definition: Ischemic strokes account for most (about 80-85%) stroke cases. These occur when a blood vessel supplying the brain becomes obstructed, typically due to a blood clot or the build-up of fatty deposits known as plaques. The lack of blood flow starves brain cells of oxygen and nutrients, leading to cellular damage and potentially irreversible consequences.

• Subtypes:

• Thrombotic Stroke: Arising from the formation of a blood clot within a blood vessel supplying the brain.

• Embolic Stroke: Occurs when a blood clot forms elsewhere in the body and travels to the brain, causing an obstruction.

• Risk Factors: Conditions such as atherosclerosis, hypertension, and diabetes contribute to the development of ischemic strokes.

2. Hemorrhagic Stroke:

• Definition: Hemorrhagic strokes, though less common, are often more severe. They result from the rupture of a blood vessel within the brain, leading to bleeding into the surrounding tissues. The increased pressure can cause significant damage to brain cells and impair neurological function.

• Subtypes:

• Intracerebral Hemorrhage: Bleeding occurs within the brain tissue, usually from small arteries damaged by conditions like hypertension.

• Subarachnoid Hemorrhage: Involving bleeding into the space surrounding the brain, often caused by the rupture of an aneurysm.

• Risk Factors: Conditions that weaken blood vessels, such as hypertension and aneurysms, elevate the risk of hemorrhagic strokes.

Distinguishing Features:

• Onset and Symptoms: Ischemic strokes often have a more gradual onset, while hemorrhagic strokes may manifest suddenly with severe symptoms.

• Severity: Hemorrhagic strokes tend to be more severe, and the outcomes can be influenced by the extent of bleeding and its location.

Prevention and Management:

• Ischemic Stroke: Prevention strategies often focus on managing risk factors, including lifestyle modifications and medications to control conditions like hypertension and diabetes. Acute treatment may involve the use of clot-busting drugs or mechanical thrombectomy.

• Hemorrhagic Stroke: Prevention addresses risk factors

and monitors conditions that could lead to vessel rupture. Treatment may include surgical intervention to repair aneurysms or control bleeding.

STROKE RISK FACTORS

Stroke, a complex interplay of vascular events in the brain, often emerges from a confluence of risk factors that can be both modifiable and non-modifiable. Recognizing and addressing these factors is pivotal for effective stroke prevention and management. Here are some key risk factors associated with strokes.

1. Hypertension:

• The Silent Culprit: Hypertension, or high blood pressure, stands as a silent yet potent contributor to stroke risk. Prolonged elevated blood pressure damages arteries, making them susceptible to the formation of clots or rupture, leading to ischemic or hemorrhagic strokes, respectively.

2. High Cholesterol:

• Arterial Blockades: Elevated levels of cholesterol, mainly low-density lipoprotein (LDL or "bad" cholesterol), contribute to the formation of plaques in the arteries. These plaques can rupture, causing blood clots that may travel to the brain, triggering ischemic strokes.

3. Diabetes:

• Vascular Complications: Diabetes, both Type 1 and Type 2, heightens the risk of strokes. It contributes to the development of atherosclerosis, narrowing blood vessels and increasing the likelihood of blood clots, amplifying the risk of ischemic strokes.

4. Smoking:

• A Hazardous Habit: Smoking not only damages blood vessels but also accelerates the progression of atherosclerosis. Additionally, it promotes blood clot formation, making smokers more susceptible to both ischemic and hemorrhagic strokes.

5. Age and Gender:

• The Influence of Time: Advancing age is a non-modifiable risk factor, with the likelihood of strokes increasing as individuals grow older. Moreover, stroke risk differs between genders, with women facing increased risk due to factors such as hormonal fluctuations and longer life expectancy.

6. Family History:

• Genetic Threads: A family history of stroke or cardiovascular diseases can elevate an individual's risk. While genetics play a role, shared lifestyle factors within families can also contribute to this heightened risk.

7. Previous Stroke or Transient Ischemic Attack (TIA):

• Warning Signs: Individuals with a history of stroke or transient ischemic attack (TIA), often referred to as a "mini-stroke," are at an increased risk of subsequent strokes. TIAs serve as warning signs, indicating an underlying vascular issue that requires attention.

Mitigation and Prevention:

• Lifestyle Modifications: Adopting a heart-healthy lifestyle, including regular physical activity, a balanced diet, and weight management, can mitigate many of these risk factors.

• Medication Adherence: For conditions like hypertension, high cholesterol, and diabetes, adherence to prescribed medications is crucial for maintaining optimal vascular health.

• Smoking Cessation: Quitting smoking significantly reduces stroke risk and improves overall cardiovascular health.

CAUSES OF STROKE

A stroke, a formidable force within the realm of cardiovascular events, unfolds as a consequence of intricate interplays of factors that can originate from both within the body and external influences. Understanding the diverse causes of stroke is paramount for effective prevention, timely intervention, and the subsequent management of this potentially life-altering event.

1. Ischemic Causes:

• Atherosclerosis: The gradual accumulation of fatty deposits or plaques within blood vessels can lead to atherosclerosis. These plaques can rupture, triggering blood clot formation that may subsequently obstruct blood flow to the brain—a hallmark of ischemic strokes.

• Embolism: Blood clots formed in distant parts of the body, such as the heart, can travel through the bloodstream and lodge in the brain's arteries, causing an embolic stroke.

• Small Vessel Disease: Damage to the small blood vessels within the brain, often associated with conditions like hypertension and diabetes, can contribute to lacunar strokes, a subtype of ischemic strokes.

2. Hemorrhagic Causes:

• Hypertension: Prolonged high blood pressure can

weaken and rupture blood vessels within the brain, leading to hemorrhagic strokes. This is particularly common in conditions of long-standing, uncontrolled hypertension.

• Aneurysms: Weakened areas in blood vessel walls, known as aneurysms, may rupture and spill blood into the brain, causing hemorrhagic strokes.

• Arteriovenous Malformations (AVMs): Abnormal connections between arteries and veins, present from birth, can disrupt normal blood flow and contribute to the risk of bleeding within the brain.

3. Other Contributing Factors:

• Medical Conditions: Certain medical conditions, including atrial fibrillation (an irregular heart rhythm) and autoimmune disorders, can increase the likelihood of blood clots and, subsequently, ischemic strokes.

• Genetic Factors: Hereditary conditions may predispose individuals to strokes. These genetic influences can impact factors such as blood clotting mechanisms and arterial structure.

• Lifestyle Factors: Unhealthy lifestyle choices, such as a diet high in saturated fats, physical inactivity, smoking, and excessive alcohol consumption, contribute to the development of risk factors like hypertension and atherosclerosis.

4. Transient Ischemic Attacks (TIAs):

• Warning Signs: Often referred to as "mini-strokes," TIAs are temporary disruptions of blood flow to the brain. While not causing permanent damage, TIAs serve as critical indicators of underlying vascular issues that may lead to more severe strokes if left unaddressed.

SYMPTOMS OF STROKE

A stroke, an abrupt disruption of blood flow to the brain, is a medical emergency demanding immediate attention. The key to minimizing its impact lies in swift recognition and prompt intervention. Understanding the symptoms of stroke is critical for individuals, caregivers, and healthcare professionals alike, as early detection can significantly improve outcomes.

1. Sudden Onset:

• Ischemic Stroke: Symptoms often develop rapidly and may worsen over minutes to hours.

• Hemorrhagic Stroke: The onset is typically sudden and severe, reflecting the rapid accumulation of blood within the brain.

2. F.A.S.T. Acronym:

• F: Face Drooping: One side of the face may droop or feel numb. Ask the person to smile and check if the smile is uneven.

• A: Arm Weakness: Arm numbness or weakness may occur. Ask the person to raise both arms and observe if one arm drifts downward.

• S: Speech Difficulty: Slurred speech, difficulty speaking, or the inability to articulate words may be present. Ask the person to repeat a simple sentence to assess speech clarity.

• T: Time to Call Emergency Services: Time is crucial. If any of these signs are observed, call emergency services immediately.

3. Other Common Symptoms:

• Sudden Severe Headache: A severe and abrupt headache, often described as the "worst headache of my life," may indicate a hemorrhagic stroke.

• Trouble Walking or Lack of Coordination: Difficulty walking, loss of balance, or lack of coordination may be observed, making everyday activities challenging.

4. Transient Ischemic Attack (TIA) Symptoms:

• Brief Episodes: TIAs, often considered warning signs, have symptoms similar to strokes but are temporary. These include sudden numbness or weakness, temporary loss of vision, and difficulty speaking.

5. Specific Symptoms Based on Stroke Location:

• Left Hemisphere Stroke: This may cause right-sided weakness or paralysis, difficulty speaking, and problems with logical thinking.

• Right Hemisphere Stroke: This may cause left-sided weakness, spatial perception issues, and difficulty recognizing faces or objects.

6. Individual Variation:

• Symptom Variability: Symptoms can vary widely among individuals, depending on the type of stroke, the affected area of the brain, and the severity of the event.

DIAGNOSIS

The diagnosis of a stroke is a time-sensitive process that involves a multifaceted approach, blending clinical evaluation, medical imaging, and detailed patient history. Rapid and accurate diagnosis is crucial for timely interventions that minimize damage and improve outcomes. Here are the critical elements in the diagnosis of stroke:

1. Clinical Evaluation:

• Medical History: A thorough assessment of the patient's medical history is crucial, including any pre-existing conditions, medications, and risk factors.

• Physical Examination: Clinical evaluation involves a detailed physical examination, with particular attention to neurological signs such as weakness, coordination, and speech abnormalities.

2. Stroke Scales:

• NIH Stroke Scale (NIHSS): A standardized scale used to assess the severity of stroke symptoms, aiding in treatment decisions and predicting outcomes.

• Glasgow Coma Scale (GCS): Evaluates a patient's level of consciousness, helping to gauge the extent of brain impairment.

3. Imaging Studies:

• CT Scan: Often the initial imaging choice, a CT scan can swiftly identify bleeding in the brain (hemorrhagic stroke) and rule out other conditions mimicking stroke symptoms.

• MRI: More detailed than a CT scan, an MRI provides a comprehensive view of brain structures and is especially useful in identifying ischemic strokes and assessing the extent of the damage.

4. Blood Tests:

• Coagulation Studies: To assess the blood's clotting ability and identify any disorders that may contribute to stroke.

• Blood Glucose Levels: Immediate assessment of blood sugar levels helps rule out conditions that mimic stroke symptoms.

5. Vascular Imaging:

• CT Angiography (CTA) and MR Angiography (MRA): These imaging techniques visualize blood vessels, identifying abnormalities such as clots or vessel narrowing.

• Carotid Ultrasound: Assesses blood flow in the carotid arteries, which is crucial for identifying potential sources of emboli.

6. Electrocardiogram (ECG or EKG):

• Heart Rhythm Assessment: Identifies irregular heart rhythms (atrial fibrillation) that may contribute to clot formation and stroke.

7. Lumbar Puncture (Spinal Tap):

• Cerebrospinal Fluid Analysis: In rare cases, a lumbar

puncture may be performed to rule out conditions that present with similar symptoms.

8. Telemedicine and Remote Diagnostics:

• Emerging Technologies: Telemedicine allows remote assessment of stroke symptoms, enabling swift consultation with stroke specialists and facilitating timely decision-making.

9. Collaboration and Team Approach:

• Multidisciplinary Care: Stroke diagnosis often involves collaboration between emergency physicians, neurologists, neuroradiologists, and other specialists to ensure a comprehensive and timely evaluation.

TREATMENT

A stroke, with its sudden and often devastating impact on the brain, demands a swift and coordinated response in its treatment. The intricacies of stroke care involve a multidisciplinary approach encompassing acute interventions, rehabilitation, and ongoing management. Here are the stroke treatments:

1. Acute Interventions:

• Intravenous Thrombolytics (Alteplase): Administered within a specific time window after symptom onset, intravenous thrombolytics work to dissolve blood clots and restore blood flow in ischemic strokes.

• Mechanical Thrombectomy: In some instances, a minimally invasive procedure involves the removal of a blood clot using specialized devices, significantly improving outcomes for eligible patients.

2. Blood Pressure Management:

• Control of Hypertension: Maintaining optimal blood pressure is crucial to prevent further damage and reduce the risk of recurrent strokes.

3. Neuroprotective Measures:

• Medications: Some medications aim to protect brain cells from damage during and after a stroke, although research in this area continues to evolve.

4. Monitoring and Supportive Care:

• Intensive Care Unit (ICU) Care: Critical for patients with severe strokes, close monitoring in an ICU setting ensures timely response to any complications.

• Oxygen Therapy: Ensures optimal oxygen levels for brain function, particularly in cases of respiratory distress.

5. Rehabilitation Services:

• Physical Therapy: Focuses on improving strength, coordination, and mobility.

• Occupational Therapy: Aims to enhance daily living skills, including self-care tasks.

• Speech Therapy: Addresses communication and swallowing difficulties often associated with strokes.

• Recreational Therapy: Engages patients in meaningful activities to enhance overall well-being.

6. Secondary Prevention:

• Medications: Antiplatelet agents, anticoagulants, and medications to control risk factors like hypertension and diabetes are often prescribed for ongoing management.

• Lifestyle Modifications: Emphasizing a heart-healthy lifestyle, including regular exercise, a balanced diet, and smoking cessation, is crucial to prevent recurrent strokes.

7. Addressing Complications:

• Management of Swallowing Difficulties: Prevents aspiration pneumonia, a common complication after strokes.

• Treatment of Depression and Emotional Support:

Critical aspects of post-stroke care, addressing the emotional impact and facilitating mental health.

8. Telemedicine and Remote Monitoring:

• Emerging Technologies: Telemedicine facilitates ongoing monitoring and follow-up care, ensuring accessibility and continuity of care, especially for patients in remote locations.

9. Research and Innovation:

• Clinical Trials: Ongoing research explores innovative therapies and treatment strategies, shaping the future of stroke care.

COMPLICATIONS

A stroke, with its sudden disruption of blood flow to the brain, can leave a profound impact, not only during the acute phase but also in the aftermath, giving rise to a spectrum of complications that influence recovery and long-term outcomes. Understanding and addressing these complications are integral components of comprehensive stroke care.

1. Physical Complications:

• Motor Weakness or Paralysis: Impaired movement or paralysis, often affecting one side of the body, is a common consequence of stroke.

• Spasticity: Increased muscle tone leading to stiffness, spasms, and difficulties with joint movement.

• Balance and Coordination Issues: Challenges in maintaining balance and coordinating movements increase the risk of falls.

2. Communication and Cognitive Complications:

• Aphasia: Impaired ability to understand or express language, affecting speaking, writing, and comprehension.

• Cognitive Impairment: Difficulties with memory, attention, problem-solving, and other cognitive functions.

3. Sensory Complications:

• Visual Impairments: Changes in vision, including blurred vision, double vision, or visual field deficits.

• Sensory Loss: Altered sensations, such as numbness or tingling, often affect one side of the body.

4. Swallowing Difficulties:

• Dysphagia: Impaired swallowing function can lead to aspiration pneumonia and malnutrition if not addressed.

5. Emotional and Psychological Complications:

• Post-Stroke Depression: Common among stroke survivors, it affects mood, motivation, and overall emotional well-being.

• Anxiety: Experiencing heightened worry or fear, often related to the challenges of recovery.

6. Cardiovascular Complications:

• Deep Vein Thrombosis (DVT) and Pulmonary Embolism (PE): Immobility after a stroke increases the risk of blood clots forming in the legs, potentially leading to DVT or PE.

• Heart Complications: Stroke can strain the heart, leading to conditions like heart failure or arrhythmias.

7. Pain and Fatigue:

• Central Post-Stroke Pain: Persistent pain, often in the arms, legs, or face, resulting from damage to the central nervous system.

• Fatigue: Overwhelming tiredness that can impact daily activities and quality of life.

8. Urinary and Bowel Complications:

• Incontinence: Difficulty controlling bladder or bowel

function may require management strategies.

9. Prevention of Recurrent Strokes:

• Secondary Prevention: Addressing risk factors like hypertension, diabetes, and high cholesterol to prevent future strokes.

10. Caregiver Strain:

• Burden on Caregivers: The demands of caregiving can lead to physical, emotional, and financial strain on family members or caregivers.

11. Post-Stroke Seizures:

• Epilepsy: Some individuals may experience seizures after a stroke, requiring appropriate management and treatment.

12. Social and Vocational Challenges:

• Social Isolation: Difficulty participating in social activities due to physical or cognitive limitations.

• Occupational Challenges: Returning to work may be challenging, requiring vocational support and adjustments.

STROKE PREVENTION

Stroke prevention is a proactive and multifaceted endeavor, encompassing lifestyle modifications, health monitoring, and risk factor management. By understanding and incorporating critical components into one's daily life, individuals can significantly reduce the risk of strokes. Here are the fundamental elements of stroke prevention:

1. Blood Pressure Management:

• Regular Monitoring: Routine blood pressure checks are essential for early detection and management of hypertension, a major stroke risk factor.

• Healthy Lifestyle Choices: Adopting a diet rich in fruits, vegetables, and whole grains, limiting sodium intake, and engaging in regular physical activity contribute to blood pressure control.

2. Healthy Diet:

• Heart-Healthy Eating: Embrace a diet low in saturated and trans fats, emphasizing fruits, vegetables, whole grains, lean proteins, and omega-3 fatty acids.

• Limiting Added Sugars and Processed Foods: Minimize the consumption of sugary beverages and processed foods high in unhealthy fats and sugars.

3. Physical Activity:

• Regular Exercise: Engage in aerobic exercises like brisk walking, jogging, or swimming for at least 150 minutes per week, along with strength training exercises twice a week.

• Maintaining a Healthy Weight: Physical activity, combined with a balanced diet, helps in weight management, reducing the risk of obesity-related conditions.

4. Smoking Cessation:

• Quitting Smoking: Smoking significantly increases stroke risk. Seeking support, such as counseling or nicotine replacement therapies, can enhance the chances of successful cessation.

5. Moderate Alcohol Consumption:

• Limiting Intake: For those who consume alcohol, moderation is key. Guidelines suggest up to one drink per day for women and up to two drinks per day for men.

6. Regular Health Check-ups:

• Comprehensive Assessment: Regular medical check-ups help monitor key health indicators, including blood pressure, cholesterol levels, and blood sugar.

• Screening for Atrial Fibrillation (AFib): Detecting and managing irregular heart rhythms, such as AFib, is crucial in stroke prevention.

7. Medication Adherence:

• Following Prescribed Medications: For individuals with conditions like hypertension, diabetes, or high cholesterol, adherence to prescribed medications is vital for effective management.

8. Diabetes Management:

• Blood Sugar Control: Monitoring blood sugar levels, adopting a balanced diet, and adhering to diabetes management plans contribute to stroke prevention.

• Lifestyle Modifications: Regular exercise and weight management play critical roles in diabetes prevention and management.

9. Stress Management:

• Mind-Body Techniques: Practices such as meditation, yoga, and deep-breathing exercises can help manage stress levels, contributing to overall cardiovascular health.

10. Sleep Hygiene:

• Adequate Sleep: Prioritize quality sleep, aiming for 7-9 hours per night. Poor sleep is associated with an increased risk of cardiovascular issues, including strokes.

11. Knowledge and Awareness:

• Recognizing Warning Signs: Being aware of the signs and symptoms of stroke enables prompt action, potentially reducing the severity of an event.

CHAPTER TWO

The role of diet in stroke prevention and recovery is pivotal, influencing vascular health and contributing to overall well-being. A stroke diet emphasizes nutrient-dense, heart-healthy foods tailored to address risk factors and support rehabilitation. Here's a comprehensive guide to understanding the principles and components of an effective stroke diet:

A. Fruits and Vegetables:

Antioxidants and Vitamins:

Purpose: Antioxidants, found abundantly in fruits and vegetables, combat oxidative stress, reduce inflammation, and protect blood vessels.

Examples: Berries (rich in anthocyanins), citrus fruits (vitamin C), and leafy greens (vitamin K) offer diverse antioxidant and vitamin profiles.

Fiber Content:

Purpose: High fiber intake supports heart health by aiding in weight management, controlling blood sugar levels, and promoting healthy digestion.

Sources: Apples, pears, broccoli, and legumes are excellent sources of dietary fiber.

B. Whole Grains:

Importance of Fiber:

Purpose: Whole grains provide essential nutrients and fiber, helping regulate blood sugar levels and contributing to heart health.

Examples: Quinoa, brown rice, oats, and whole wheat products are excellent choices.

Examples of Whole Grains:

Diversity: Incorporate a variety of whole grains for a broader range of nutrients. Examples include barley, bulgur, and farro.

C. Lean Proteins:

Fish and Omega-3 Fatty Acids:

Purpose: Fatty fish like salmon and mackerel provide omega-3 fatty acids, which have anti-inflammatory effects and support heart health.

Frequency: Aim for at least two servings of fatty fish per week.

Poultry, Beans, and Legumes:

Purpose: Lean proteins from sources like poultry, beans, and legumes contribute to muscle health and provide essential nutrients.

Diversity: Incorporate a mix of plant-based and lean animal-based proteins for variety and nutritional balance.

D. Healthy Fats:

Monounsaturated and Polyunsaturated Fats:

Purpose: These heart-healthy fats help reduce LDL cholesterol levels and support overall cardiovascular health.

Sources: Olive oil, avocados, and nuts are rich in monounsaturated fats, while fatty fish, flaxseeds, and walnuts provide polyunsaturated fats.

Sources of Healthy Fats:

Inclusion: Include a variety of sources in your diet, such as seeds, chia seeds, and fatty fish, to ensure a diverse intake of beneficial fats.

E. Sodium Control:

Impact of High Sodium on Blood Pressure:

Connection: High sodium intake is linked to elevated blood pressure, a significant risk factor for strokes.

Awareness: Be vigilant about hidden sources of sodium in processed foods and restaurant meals.

Tips for Reducing Sodium Intake:

Fresh Food Choices: Prioritize fresh, whole foods over processed options.

• Spice It Up: Use herbs, spices, and alternative seasonings to enhance flavor without relying on excessive salt.

F. Alcohol Moderation:

Recommended Limits:

Guidelines: Moderation is key—up to one drink per day for women and up to two drinks per day for men.

Awareness: Understand and adhere to recommended limits to mitigate potential risks.

Risks Associated with Excessive Alcohol Consumption:

• Stroke Risk: Excessive alcohol intake is associated with an increased risk of stroke and other cardiovascular issues.

• Health Considerations: Be mindful of individual health conditions and make informed decisions about alcohol consumption.

G. Hydration:

Importance of Water in Stroke Prevention:

• Hydration Benefits: Proper hydration supports overall health, aiding in digestion, circulation, and temperature regulation.

• Water as a Primary Beverage: Choose water as the primary beverage, limiting sugary drinks and excessive caffeine intake.

Recommendations for Staying Hydrated:

• Regular Intake: Consume water throughout the day, especially during meals and physical activity.

• Monitoring Urine Color: A pale yellow urine color indicates adequate hydration.

IMPORTANCE OF A HEALTHY DIET

A healthy diet stands as a cornerstone of overall well-being, influencing physical health, mental clarity, and longevity. It is not merely a means of weight management but a powerful tool that shapes the body's resilience against diseases and contributes to a vibrant and energetic life. Here are the importance of a healthy diet:

1. Disease Prevention:

• Cardiovascular Health: A heart-healthy diet rich in fruits, vegetables, whole grains, and lean proteins helps prevent conditions like hypertension and atherosclerosis.

• Type 2 Diabetes: Balanced nutrition, focusing on complex carbohydrates and portion control, plays a crucial role in preventing and managing diabetes.

• Cancer Prevention: Certain dietary choices, such as consuming antioxidant-rich foods, may contribute to reducing the risk of certain cancers.

2. Weight Management:

• Body Composition: A nutritious diet supports a healthy body weight, reducing the risk of obesity-related conditions like heart disease and joint problems.

• Metabolic Health: Balanced nutrition helps regulate metabolism, fostering a sustainable and energy-efficient physiological state.

3. Cognitive Function:

• Brain Health: Nutrients like omega-3 fatty acids, antioxidants, and vitamins support cognitive function, memory, and concentration.

• Reduced Cognitive Decline: A diet rich in fruits, vegetables, and whole grains may contribute to a lower risk of age-related cognitive decline.

4. Energy and Vitality:

• Nutrient-rich foods: Proper nutrition ensures a steady energy supply, supporting daily activities and exercise.

• Blood Sugar Stability: Balanced meals and snacks contribute to stable blood sugar levels, preventing energy crashes and fatigue.

5. Gastrointestinal Health:

• Fiber Intake: Adequate fiber from fruits, vegetables, and whole grains supports digestive health and helps prevent conditions like constipation.

• Microbiome Balance: A diverse and balanced diet promotes a healthy gut microbiome, which is crucial for overall gastrointestinal well-being.

6. Bone Health:

• Calcium and Vitamin D: Essential for bone health, these nutrients are found in dairy products, leafy greens, and exposure to sunlight.

• Reduced Osteoporosis Risk: A diet supporting optimal bone health can reduce the risk of osteoporosis and fractures.

7. Immune Function:

• Nutrient-Rich Foods: Essential nutrients like vitamins C and D, zinc, and antioxidants support a robust immune system.

• Reduced Susceptibility to Infections: A well-nourished body is better equipped to fend off infections and recover efficiently.

8. Mental Health:

• Omega-3 Fatty Acids: Found in fish, flaxseeds, and walnuts, these contribute to mental well-being and may reduce the risk of depression.

• Balanced Blood Sugar: Stable blood sugar levels from a balanced diet help regulate mood and reduce irritability.

9. Longevity and Quality of Life:

• Disease Prevention: A healthy diet is linked to a lower risk of chronic diseases, contributing to a longer and higher quality of life.

• Physical and Mental Well-Being: Optimal nutrition supports physical and mental resilience, enhancing the ability to enjoy life's experiences.

10. Sustainable Lifestyle Habits:

• Lifelong Habits: Establishing healthy eating patterns early in life fosters habits that can be sustained throughout adulthood.

• Prevention of Lifestyle-Related Diseases: A well-balanced diet plays a crucial role in preventing diseases associated with sedentary lifestyles and poor dietary choices.

SAMPLE MEAL PLAN

Creating a stroke-preventive meal plan involves a careful selection of nutrient-dense foods that support cardiovascular health, manage risk factors, and contribute to overall well-being. Below is a sample meal plan for several days, designed to showcase variety, balance, and adherence to dietary principles associated with stroke prevention.

DAY 1:

Breakfast:

• Oatmeal topped with fresh berries and a sprinkle of chia seeds.

• A small handful of walnuts for added omega-3 fatty acids.

• Green tea or black coffee.

Lunch:

• Grilled chicken breast salad with mixed greens, cherry tomatoes, cucumber, and a vinaigrette dressing.

• Quinoa or brown rice on the side for whole grains.

• A piece of fresh fruit for dessert.

Dinner:

• Baked salmon with a lemon and herb marinade.

• Steamed broccoli and carrots as side vegetables.

• Sweet potato wedges are a complex carbohydrate source.

Snack:

• Greek yogurt with a drizzle of honey and a handful of almonds.

DAY 2:

Breakfast:

• Whole grain toast with avocado spread and poached eggs.

• A fruit smoothie with spinach, banana, and a splash of almond milk.

Lunch:

• Lentil soup with a side of whole-grain crackers.

• Mixed vegetable stir-fry with tofu or lean chicken.

• Sliced oranges for dessert.

Dinner:

• Quinoa-stuffed bell peppers with lean ground turkey and black beans.

• Grilled zucchini and asparagus on the side.

• A small serving of mixed berries for a sweet finish.

Snack:

• Carrot and cucumber sticks with hummus.

DAY 3:

Breakfast:

• Whole grain cereal with skim milk and sliced strawberries.

• A handful of pistachios for added healthy fats.

• Green tea or herbal tea.

Lunch:

• Turkey and avocado wrap with whole-grain tortilla.

• Spinach and arugula salad with a light balsamic vinaigrette.

• Apple slices for a refreshing touch.

Dinner:

• Baked cod with a lemon and garlic marinade.

• Quinoa pilaf with mixed vegetables.

• Steamed green beans as a side.

Snack:

• Cottage cheese with pineapple chunks.

DAY 4:

Breakfast:

• Smoothie bowl with blended acai, banana, mixed berries, and granola.

• A sprinkle of flaxseeds for added fiber.

Lunch:

• Chickpea salad with cherry tomatoes, cucumbers, feta cheese, and a lemon-tahini dressing.

• Whole grain pita bread on the side.

• A small bunch of grapes for dessert.

Dinner:

• Stir-fried shrimp with broccoli, bell peppers, and snap peas.

• Brown rice as a base.

• Sliced mango for a sweet and tropical touch.

Snack:

• A handful of mixed nuts (almonds, walnuts, and pistachios).

DAY 5:

Breakfast:

• Whole grain pancakes topped with sliced bananas and a drizzle of pure maple syrup.

• A cup of low-fat milk or a dairy-free alternative.

• Green tea or black coffee.

Lunch:

• Spinach and feta omelet with cherry tomatoes.

• Quinoa salad with cucumber, red onion, and a lemon herb dressing.

• Orange slices for dessert.

Dinner:

• Grilled chicken breast with rosemary and garlic.

• Roasted sweet potatoes and Brussels sprouts.

• Mixed berry parfait with Greek yogurt for dessert.

Snack:

• Sliced pear with a small serving of cheese.

DAY 6:

Breakfast:

• Avocado and smoked salmon on whole grain toast.

• Freshly squeezed orange juice.

Lunch:

• Whole wheat wrap with hummus, roasted vegetables, and grilled tofu.

• Mixed greens salad with a light vinaigrette.

• A small bunch of grapes for dessert.

Dinner:

• Baked tilapia with a mango salsa.

• Quinoa and black bean bowl with diced avocado.

• Steamed broccoli on the side.

Snack:

• A smoothie with spinach, pineapple, banana, and almond milk.

DAY 7:

Breakfast:

• Greek yogurt parfait with granola, mixed berries, and a drizzle of honey.

• Green tea or herbal tea.

Lunch:

• Turkey and vegetable kebabs with a quinoa and parsley salad.

• Sliced watermelon for a refreshing finish.

Dinner:

• Stir-fried tofu with bok choy, bell peppers, and snow peas.

• Brown rice or cauliflower rice.

• Sliced kiwi for dessert.

Snack:

• Cottage cheese with sliced peaches.

CHAPTER THREE

Fruits and Vegetables Recipes

Grilled Vegetable Salad

Meal Description: This Grilled Vegetable Salad is a celebration of vibrant colors, robust flavors, and wholesome goodness. Packed with nutrient-rich ingredients, this salad offers a delightful combination of grilled zucchini, bell peppers, cherry tomatoes, and red onions, drizzled with light, tangy olive oil and balsamic vinegar dressing. The infusion of herbs adds an aromatic touch, creating a refreshing and satisfying dish that is perfect for a light lunch or a flavorful side.

Ingredients:

• Two zucchinis, sliced lengthwise

• One red bell pepper, cut into strips

• One yellow bell pepper, cut into strips

• 1 cup cherry tomatoes, halved

• One red onion, thinly sliced

• Two tablespoons of olive oil

• Three tablespoons balsamic vinegar

• One teaspoon of dried herbs (such as oregano, thyme, or Italian seasoning)

• Salt and pepper to taste

Step-by-Step Instructions:

Preheat the Grill:

• Preheat your grill to medium-high heat.

Prepare the Vegetables:

• Toss the sliced zucchini, bell peppers, cherry tomatoes,

and red onions with olive oil, balsamic vinegar, dried herbs, salt, and pepper in a large bowl.

Grill the Vegetables:

• Place the marinated vegetables on the preheated grill.

• Grill for 5-7 minutes, turning occasionally, until the vegetables have grill marks and are tender but still slightly crisp.

Assemble the Salad:

• Transfer the grilled vegetables to a serving platter or bowl.

• Drizzle any remaining marinade from the bowl over the vegetables.

Serve:

• Serve the Grilled Vegetable Salad warm or at room temperature.

Nutrition Information (Per Serving):

• Calories: 180 calories

• Protein: 4g

• Fat: 12g

• Carbohydrates: 18g

• Fiber: 5g

• Sugar: 10g

• Sodium: 120mg

FRUIT SMOOTHIE BOWL

Meal Description: This Fruit Smoothie Bowl is a delightful fusion of vibrant berries, creamy bananas, nutrient-packed spinach, velvety Greek yogurt, and the nutty goodness of almond milk. Topped with chia seeds for added texture and nutritional benefits, this smoothie bowl is a treat for taste buds and a powerhouse of vitamins, minerals, and antioxidants. Perfect for breakfast or a refreshing snack, it's a delicious way to kickstart your day with a burst of energy.

Ingredients:

• 1 cup mixed berries (strawberries, blueberries, raspberries)

• One ripe banana, frozen

• 1 cup fresh spinach leaves

• 1/2 cup Greek yogurt

• 1/2 cup unsweetened almond milk

• One tablespoon of chia seeds

Toppings (Optional):

• Sliced strawberries

• Blueberries

- Granola

- Coconut flakes

- Drizzle of honey

Step-by-Step Instructions:

Prepare the Base:

• Combine the mixed berries, frozen banana, fresh spinach, Greek yogurt, and almond milk in a blender.

Blend Until Smooth:

• Blend the ingredients until smooth and creamy. If the mixture is too thick, you can add more almond milk in small increments until you reach your desired consistency.

Assemble the Smoothie Bowl:

• Pour the smoothie into a bowl.

Add Toppings:

• Sprinkle chia seeds on top for added texture and nutritional benefits.

• Arrange sliced strawberries, blueberries, granola, and coconut flakes as desired.

Drizzle with Honey (Optional):

• Drizzle a small amount of honey over the toppings for a touch of sweetness.

Enjoy Immediately:

• Grab a spoon and enjoy your delicious and nutritious Fruit Smoothie Bowl immediately.

Nutrition Information (Per Serving):

• Calories: 280 calories

- Protein: 12g
- Fat: 8g
- Carbohydrates: 45g
- Fiber: 10g
- Sugar: 24g
- Sodium: 90mg

STUFFED BELL PEPPERS

Meal Description: These Stuffed Bell Peppers are a culinary masterpiece, blending the nutty richness of quinoa, the heartiness of black beans, the sweetness of corn, and the savory notes of tomatoes and onions. Seasoned with a medley of spices, each bite is a delightful explosion of flavors. Topped with creamy avocado, these stuffed peppers satisfy your taste buds and provide a wholesome and balanced meal. Perfect for lunch or dinner, this dish is a celebration of nutritious ingredients presented in a vibrant and colorful package.

Ingredients:

• Four large bell peppers, halved and seeds removed

• 1 cup cooked quinoa

• 1 cup black beans, canned or cooked

• 1 cup corn kernels (fresh or frozen)

• 1 cup diced tomatoes

• 1/2 cup diced onions

• One teaspoon cumin

• One teaspoon of chili powder

• 1/2 teaspoon garlic powder

• Salt and pepper to taste

• One avocado, sliced (for topping)

Optional Garnishes:

• Fresh cilantro

• Lime wedges

Step-by-Step Instructions:

Preheat the Oven:

• Preheat your oven to 375°F (190°C).

Prepare the Bell Peppers:

• Cut the bell peppers in half lengthwise and remove the seeds and membranes.

Prepare the Filling:

• Mix cooked quinoa, black beans, corn, tomatoes, diced onions, cumin, chili powder, garlic powder, salt, and pepper in a large bowl.

Stuff the Peppers:

• Spoon the quinoa and vegetable mixture into each bell pepper half, pressing down gently to pack the filling.

Bake:

• Place the stuffed bell peppers in a baking dish.

• Bake in the preheated oven for 25-30 minutes or until the peppers are tender.

Top with Avocado:

• Once out of the oven, top each stuffed pepper with slices of fresh avocado.

Garnish and Serve:

• Garnish with fresh cilantro and serve with lime wedges on the side.

Nutrition Information (Per Serving - 2 halves):

• Calories: 320 calories

• Protein: 10g

• Fat: 10g

• Carbohydrates: 50g

• Fiber: 12g

• Sugar: 7g

• Sodium: 240mg

MANGO AVOCADO SALSA

Meal Description: This Mango Avocado Salsa is a harmonious blend of vibrant colors and fresh flavors, creating a taste sensation that transports you to a tropical paradise. Juicy mangoes, creamy avocados, zesty red onions, and aromatic cilantro dance together in perfect rhythm, while a splash of lime juice and a pinch of salt enhance the symphony. Whether served as a topping for grilled chicken or fish or enjoyed with tortilla chips, this salsa is a celebration of simplicity and exquisite taste, making every bite a refreshing delight.

Ingredients:

• Two ripe mangoes, diced

• Two avocados, diced

• 1/2 cup red onion, finely chopped

• 1/4 cup fresh cilantro, chopped

• Juice of 2 limes

• Salt to taste

Optional Additions:

• Jalapeño, finely chopped (for a hint of spice)

• Cherry tomatoes, diced (for extra freshness)

Step-by-Step Instructions:

Prepare the Mango and Avocado:

• Peel and dice the ripe mangoes and avocados.

Chop the Vegetables:

• Finely chop the red onion and fresh cilantro.

Combine Ingredients:

• In a mixing bowl, gently combine the diced mangoes, avocados, chopped red onion, and cilantro.

Add Lime Juice:

• Squeeze the juice of two limes over the mixture.

Season with Salt:

• Sprinkle salt to taste and gently toss the ingredients until well combined.

Optional Additions:

• If you prefer a bit of heat, add finely chopped jalapeño.

• For extra freshness, consider adding diced cherry tomatoes.

Chill (Optional):

• Allow the salsa to chill in the refrigerator for about 30 minutes to let the flavors meld.

Serve and Enjoy:

• Serve the Mango Avocado Salsa as a topping for grilled proteins or as a refreshing dip with tortilla chips.

Nutrition Information (Per Serving):

• Calories: 120 calories

• Protein: 2g

- Fat: 8g
- Carbohydrates: 15g
- Fiber: 6g
- Sugar: 8g
- Sodium: 200mg

ROASTED BRUSSELS SPROUTS

Meal Description: These Roasted Brussels Sprouts are a culinary revelation, transforming humble Brussels sprouts into a crispy and flavorful dish. Tossed in olive oil, minced garlic, and lemon zest, the sprouts undergo a magical transformation in the oven. The result is a medley of textures—crispy on the outside and tender on the inside—enhanced by the citrusy zing of lemon. Whether served as a side dish or a snack, these roasted Brussels sprouts are a testament to the art of simple, delicious cooking.

Ingredients:

• 1 pound Brussels sprouts, trimmed and halved

• Two tablespoons of olive oil

• Three cloves garlic, minced

• Zest of 1 lemon

• Salt and pepper to taste

Optional Additions:

• Grated Parmesan cheese (for a savory kick)

• Balsamic glaze (for a sweet and tangy finish)

Step-by-Step Instructions:

Preheat the Oven:

• Preheat your oven to 400°F (200°C).

Prepare Brussels Sprouts:

• Trim the Brussels sprouts, removing any outer leaves that are wilted or brown. Cut them in half.

Prepare the Seasoning:

• Combine the halved Brussels sprouts in a bowl with olive oil, minced garlic, lemon zest, salt, and pepper. Toss until the Brussels sprouts are evenly coated.

Arrange on Baking Sheet:

• Spread the seasoned Brussels sprouts in a single layer on a baking sheet.

Roast in the Oven:

• Roast in the preheated oven for 25-30 minutes or until the Brussels sprouts are golden brown and crispy on the edges.

Optional Additions:

• If desired, sprinkle grated Parmesan cheese over the roasted Brussels sprouts during the last 5 minutes of baking.

• Drizzle with balsamic glaze before serving for an extra layer of flavor.

Serve Hot:

• Transfer the roasted Brussels sprouts to a serving dish and serve hot.

Nutrition Information (Per Serving):

- Calories: 120 calories
- Protein: 4g
- Fat: 7g
- Carbohydrates: 14g
- Fiber: 6g
- Sugar: 3g
- Sodium: 40mg

CUCUMBER AND TOMATO SALAD

Meal Description: This Cucumber and Tomato Salad is a refreshing and vibrant combination of crisp cucumbers, juicy tomatoes, zesty red onions, briny olives, and creamy feta cheese, all brought together with a drizzle of extra-virgin olive oil. Inspired by Mediterranean flavors, this salad is a celebration of simplicity, allowing the natural freshness of the ingredients to shine. Perfect as a light side dish or a standalone salad, it's a culinary journey to the sun-soaked coasts of the Mediterranean.

Ingredients:

- Two cucumbers, sliced

- 2 cups cherry tomatoes, halved

- 1/2 red onion, thinly sliced

- 1/2 cup feta cheese, crumbled

- 1/3 cup Kalamata olives, pitted and halved

- Three tablespoons extra-virgin olive oil

- Salt and pepper to taste

Optional Additions:

- Fresh oregano or basil (for additional herbaceous notes)

- Balsamic glaze (for a touch of sweetness)

Step-by-Step Instructions:

Prepare the Vegetables:

• Slice the cucumbers, halve the cherry tomatoes, and thinly slice the red onion.

Assemble the Salad:

• Combine the sliced cucumbers, halved cherry tomatoes, sliced red onion, crumbled feta cheese, and halved Kalamata olives in a large bowl.

Drizzle with Olive Oil:

• Drizzle extra-virgin olive oil over the salad.

Season to Taste:

• Season with salt and pepper to taste. Toss the salad gently to ensure an even coating.

Optional Additions:

• If desired, sprinkle fresh oregano or basil over the salad for added herbaceous flavor.

• Drizzle with balsamic glaze for a touch of sweetness and depth.

Chill (Optional):

• Allow the salad to chill in the refrigerator for about 15-30 minutes to enhance the flavors.

Serve and Enjoy:

• Serve the Cucumber and Tomato Salad as a refreshing side dish or a standalone salad.

Nutrition Information (Per Serving):

• Calories: 180 calories

• Protein: 4g

- Fat: 15g
- Carbohydrates: 10g
- Fiber: 3g
- Sugar: 5g
- Sodium: 350mg

BERRY SPINACH SALAD

Meal Description: The Berry Spinach Salad is a vibrant ensemble of nutrient-packed spinach, luscious mixed berries, creamy feta cheese, crunchy walnuts, and a drizzle of balsamic vinaigrette. This salad is a visual delight with its medley of colors and a nutritional powerhouse, combining the goodness of leafy greens with the sweetness of berries and the savory notes of feta. Whether enjoyed as a light lunch or a refreshing side, this salad is a perfect ode to the harmony of wholesome ingredients.

Ingredients:

• 6 cups fresh spinach leaves, washed and dried

• 1 cup mixed berries (strawberries, blueberries, raspberries)

• 1/2 cup feta cheese, crumbled

• 1/3 cup walnuts, chopped

• Balsamic vinaigrette (store-bought or homemade)

Optional Additions:

• Sliced red onions (for a touch of zing)

• Grilled chicken or shrimp (for added protein)

Step-by-Step Instructions:

Prepare the Spinach:

• Wash and dry the fresh spinach leaves thoroughly.

Assemble the Salad:

• Combine the fresh spinach leaves, mixed berries, crumbled feta cheese, and chopped walnuts in a large salad bowl.

Optional Additions:

• If desired, add sliced red onions for an additional burst of flavor.

Drizzle with Balsamic Vinaigrette:

• Drizzle the salad with balsamic vinaigrette, starting with a modest amount and adding more to taste.

Toss Gently:

• Toss the salad gently to ensure even distribution of the ingredients and dressing.

Optional Protein Addition:

• For a heartier version, consider adding grilled chicken or shrimp.

Serve and Enjoy:

• Serve the Berry Spinach Salad immediately, allowing everyone to enjoy the freshness of the ingredients.

Nutrition Information (Per Serving):

• Calories: 220 calories

• Protein: 8g

• Fat: 16g

• Carbohydrates: 16g

- Fiber: 5g
- Sugar: 7g
- Sodium: 250mg

VEGGIE STIR-FRY

Meal Description: This Veggie Stir-Fry is a celebration of vibrant colors and wholesome goodness, featuring crisp broccoli, sweet bell peppers, carrots, snap peas, and tofu, all bathed in a savory soy sauce glaze. Bursting with freshness and nutrition, this stir-fry is a delightful way to enjoy a medley of vegetables and plant-based protein. Quick to prepare and full of flavor, it's the perfect go-to dish for a quick and satisfying weeknight dinner.

Ingredients:

- 2 cups broccoli florets

- One red bell pepper, thinly sliced

- One yellow bell pepper, thinly sliced

- 1 cup carrots, julienned

- 1 cup snap peas, ends trimmed

- 14 oz (400g) firm tofu, cubed

- Three tablespoons soy sauce

- Two tablespoons of vegetable oil

- One teaspoon of ginger, minced

- Two cloves garlic, minced

- Sesame seeds for garnish (optional)

- Green onions, sliced (optional)

Optional Additions:

• Sliced mushrooms

• Water chestnuts

• Baby corn

Step-by-Step Instructions:

Prepare the Tofu:

• Press the tofu to remove excess water and cut it into cubes.

Heat the Pan:

• Heat vegetable oil in a large wok or skillet over medium-high heat.

Sauté Tofu:

• Add the tofu cubes and cook until golden brown on all sides. Remove from the pan and set aside.

Stir-Fry Vegetables:

• In the same pan, add a bit more oil if needed. Add minced ginger and garlic, stir briefly, then add broccoli, bell peppers, carrots, and snap peas.

Cook Vegetables:

• Stir-fry the vegetables until they are crisp-tender, retaining their vibrant colors.

Combine Tofu and Vegetables:

• Add the cooked tofu back into the pan with the vegetables.

Soy Sauce Glaze:

• Pour soy sauce over the tofu and vegetables. Toss everything to combine and allow the flavors to meld.

Garnish and Serve:

• Garnish with sesame seeds and sliced green onions if desired.

Serve Hot:

• Serve the Veggie Stir-Fry hot over rice or noodles.

Nutrition Information (Per Serving):

• Calories: 280 calories

• Protein: 18g

• Fat: 18g

• Carbohydrates: 20g

• Fiber: 7g

• Sugar: 7g

• Sodium: 900mg

GRILLED ASPARAGUS WITH LEMON

Meal Description: This Grilled Asparagus with Lemon is a simple yet elegant dish that showcases the natural flavors of fresh asparagus enhanced by the zesty brightness of lemon. Tender asparagus spears are lightly grilled to perfection and then tossed with a vibrant mixture of olive oil, lemon juice, garlic, and a pinch of salt. The result is a side dish that is visually appealing and a refreshing and delightful addition to any meal, offering a burst of citrusy goodness with every bite.

Ingredients:

• One bunch of asparagus, trimmed

• Two tablespoons of olive oil

• Two tablespoons of lemon juice (freshly squeezed)

• Two cloves garlic, minced

• Salt to taste

• Lemon zest (optional, for garnish)

Optional Additions:

• Freshly ground black pepper

• Grated Parmesan cheese

Step-by-Step Instructions:

Prepare the Asparagus:

• Trim the tough ends of the asparagus spears.

Preheat the Grill:

• Preheat a grill or grill pan over medium-high heat.

Make the Marinade:

• Whisk together olive oil, freshly squeezed lemon juice, minced garlic, and a pinch of salt in a small bowl.

Grill the Asparagus:

• Brush the asparagus spears with the marinade, ensuring they are well-coated.

• Grill the asparagus for 3-5 minutes, turning occasionally, until they are tender and have grill marks.

Transfer and Toss:

• Transfer the grilled asparagus to a serving plate.

• Drizzle any remaining marinade over the asparagus and toss gently to coat.

Optional Garnishes:

• Sprinkle with additional salt to taste.

• Garnish with lemon zest for an extra citrusy aroma.

Optional Additions:

• For added flavor, sprinkle with freshly ground black pepper or grated Parmesan cheese.

Serve Hot:

• Serve the Grilled Asparagus with Lemon hot as a

delightful side dish.

Nutrition Information (Per Serving):

• Calories: 90 calories

• Protein: 3g

• Fat: 7g

• Carbohydrates: 7g

• Fiber: 3g

• Sugar: 2g

• Sodium: 150mg

WATERMELON FETA SALAD

Meal Description: This Watermelon Feta Salad is a celebration of summer's bounty, combining the juicy sweetness of watermelon with the creamy saltiness of feta cheese, all brightened by the zesty freshness of mint and lime juice. It's a delightful balance of flavors and textures that captures the essence of summer in every bite. Perfect as a light and refreshing side dish for picnics, barbecues, or any summer gathering, this salad is a testament to the simple joys of seasonal ingredients.

Ingredients:

• 4 cups watermelon, cubed

• 1 cup feta cheese, crumbled

• 1/4 cup fresh mint leaves, chopped

• Juice of 2 limes

Optional Additions:

• Balsamic glaze (for a sweet and tangy finish)

• Sliced cucumber (for added crunch)

Step-by-Step Instructions:

Prepare the Watermelon:

• Cut the watermelon into bite-sized cubes.

Assemble the Salad:

• Combine the watermelon cubes, crumbled feta cheese, and chopped mint leaves in a large bowl.

Add Lime Juice:

• Squeeze the juice of two limes over the salad.

Toss Gently:

• Gently toss the ingredients until the watermelon, feta, and mint are evenly coated with lime juice.

Optional Additions:

• If desired, drizzle balsamic glaze over the salad for a sweet and tangy finish.

• Add sliced cucumber for an extra layer of freshness and crunch.

Chill (Optional):

• Allow the salad to chill in the refrigerator for about 15-30 minutes to enhance the flavors.

Serve and Enjoy:

• Serve the Watermelon Feta Salad as a refreshing or light summer snack.

Nutrition Information (Per Serving):

• Calories: 150 calories

• Protein: 6g

• Fat: 8g

• Carbohydrates: 18g

• Fiber: 2g

• Sugar: 14g

- Sodium: 300mg

CHAPTER FOUR

Whole Grains Recipes

Quinoa and Vegetable Stuffed Peppers

Meal Description: These Quinoa and Vegetable Stuffed Peppers are a wholesome and satisfying fusion of fluffy quinoa, protein-rich black beans, sweet corn, diced tomatoes, onions, and a medley of spices, all enveloped in colorful bell peppers. Baked to perfection, each bite is a symphony of textures and flavors—a nutritious feast that not only pleases the palate but also nourishes the body. Whether served as a standalone meal or as a hearty side, these stuffed peppers are a delicious way to embrace the goodness of plant-based ingredients.

Ingredients:

• Four large bell peppers, halved and seeds removed

• 1 cup quinoa, cooked

• 1 cup black beans, canned or cooked

• 1 cup corn kernels (fresh or frozen)

• 1 cup diced tomatoes

• 1/2 cup diced onions

• One teaspoon cumin

• One teaspoon of chili powder

• 1/2 teaspoon garlic powder

• Salt and pepper to taste

• Olive oil for drizzling

Optional Additions:

• Shredded cheese (for topping)

• Avocado slices (for garnish)

Step-by-Step Instructions:

Preheat the Oven:

• Preheat your oven to 375°F (190°C).

Prepare the Bell Peppers:

• Cut the bell peppers in half lengthwise and remove the seeds and membranes.

Prepare the Filling:

• Mix cooked quinoa, black beans, corn, tomatoes, diced onions, cumin, chili powder, garlic powder, salt, and pepper in a large bowl.

Stuff the Peppers:

• Spoon the quinoa and vegetable mixture into each bell pepper half, pressing down gently to pack the filling.

Drizzle with Olive Oil:

• Drizzle a bit of olive oil over the stuffed peppers to enhance the roasting process.

Bake:

• Place the stuffed bell peppers in a baking dish.

• Bake in the preheated oven for 25-30 minutes or until the peppers are tender.

Optional Toppings:

• If desired, sprinkle shredded cheese over the stuffed peppers during the last 5 minutes of baking.

Garnish and Serve:

• Garnish with avocado slices and fresh herbs if desired.

Nutrition Information (Per Serving - 2 halves):

• Calories: 320 calories

- Protein: 12g
- Fat: 10g
- Carbohydrates: 50g
- Fiber: 12g
- Sugar: 7g
- Sodium: 240mg

BROWN RICE BOWL WITH VEGETABLES

Meal Description: This Brown Rice Bowl with Vegetables is a nourishing and versatile dish that brings together the earthy goodness of brown rice, a colorful assortment of mixed vegetables, and your choice of protein—either tofu for a plant-based option or grilled chicken for those who prefer meat. Drizzled with savory soy sauce, this bowl is a feast for the taste buds and a balanced and nutritious meal that provides a spectrum of essential nutrients. Easy to customize and quick to prepare, it's a go-to recipe for a satisfying lunch or dinner.

Ingredients:

• 2 cups cooked brown rice

• 2 cups mixed vegetables (broccoli, bell peppers, carrots, snap peas, etc.)

• 1 cup tofu, cubed or grilled chicken, sliced

• Two tablespoons of soy sauce

• One tablespoon of vegetable oil

• Sesame seeds for garnish (optional)

• Green onions, sliced (optional)

Optional Additions:

- Sliced mushrooms

- Baby corn

- Bean sprouts

- Sriracha or chili garlic sauce (for extra heat)

Step-by-Step Instructions:

Cook Brown Rice:

- Prepare 2 cups of cooked brown rice according to package instructions.

Sauté Vegetables:

- In a large pan or wok, heat vegetable oil over medium-high heat.

- Add mixed vegetables and sauté until they are crisp-tender, retaining their vibrant colors.

Cook Protein:

- Push the vegetables to one side of the pan and add tofu or grilled chicken. Cook until tofu is lightly browned or the chicken is fully cooked.

Combine Rice and Vegetables:

- Mix the cooked brown rice with the sautéed vegetables and protein in the pan.

Drizzle with Soy Sauce:

- Pour soy sauce over the rice and vegetable mixture. Toss everything to combine and allow the flavors to meld.

Optional Additions:

- Add sliced mushrooms, baby corn, or bean sprouts for additional textures if desired.

Garnish and Serve:

• Garnish with sesame seeds and sliced green onions if desired.

Optional Heat:

• For those who enjoy some heat, drizzle with Sriracha or chili garlic sauce.

Nutrition Information (Per Serving):

• Calories: 400 calories

• Protein: 15g

• Fat: 10g

• Carbohydrates: 60g

• Fiber: 8g

• Sugar: 3g

• Sodium: 600mg

WHOLE WHEAT PASTA PRIMAVERA

Meal Description: Whole Wheat Pasta Primavera is a vibrant and wholesome dish that combines the nutty goodness of whole wheat pasta with a medley of colorful vegetables. In this recipe, al dente whole wheat pasta is tossed with crisp broccoli, sweet cherry tomatoes, and bell peppers, creating a symphony of flavors and textures. Drizzled with olive oil, this Primavera is a feast for the eyes and a nutritious celebration of seasonal vegetables. Quick to prepare and bursting with freshness, it's a perfect choice for a satisfying and healthy meal.

Ingredients:

• 2 cups whole wheat pasta, cooked

• 1 cup broccoli florets

• 1 cup cherry tomatoes, halved

• 1/2 cup bell peppers, thinly sliced

• Two tablespoons of olive oil

• Salt and pepper to taste

• Grated Parmesan cheese for garnish (optional)

• Fresh basil or parsley for garnish (optional)

Optional Additions:

- Sliced black olives

- Crushed red pepper flakes (for a touch of heat)

- Grilled chicken or shrimp (for added protein)

Step-by-Step Instructions:

Cook Whole Wheat Pasta:

- Prepare 2 cups of whole wheat pasta according to package instructions. Cook to al dente.

Steam Broccoli:

- In a separate pot, steam the broccoli florets until they are crisp-tender.

Prepare Vegetables:

- Halve the cherry tomatoes and thinly slice the bell peppers.

Toss Pasta and Vegetables:

- Combine the cooked whole wheat pasta, steamed broccoli, halved cherry tomatoes, and sliced bell peppers in a large mixing bowl.

Drizzle with Olive Oil:

- Drizzle olive oil over the pasta and vegetables. Toss everything to coat evenly.

Season to Taste:

- Season with salt and pepper to taste. Add optional crushed red pepper flakes for a hint of heat.

Optional Additions:

- For extra flavor, toss in sliced black olives.

Garnish and Serve:

- Garnish with grated Parmesan cheese and fresh basil or

parsley if desired.

Nutrition Information (Per Serving):

- Calories: Approximately 350 calories

- Protein: 12g

- Fat: 10g

- Carbohydrates: 55g

- Fiber: 8g

- Sugar: 4g

- Sodium: 200mg

BARLEY AND MUSHROOM RISOTTO

Meal Description: Barley and Mushroom Risotto offers a comforting and hearty twist to the traditional Italian dish. Nutty barley takes the place of Arborio rice, while earthy mushrooms bring a rich umami flavor. This risotto is simmered to perfection in vegetable broth, creating a creamy and satisfying dish. Finished with the savory notes of Parmesan cheese, this Barley and Mushroom Risotto is a delightful combination of textures and tastes—an ideal choice for those seeking a wholesome and substantial grain-based meal.

Ingredients:

• 1 cup barley

• 2 cups mushrooms, sliced (such as cremini or button mushrooms)

• 4 cups vegetable broth

• 1/2 cup Parmesan cheese, grated

• Two tablespoons of olive oil

• One onion, finely chopped

• Two cloves garlic, minced

• Salt and pepper to taste

• Fresh parsley for garnish (optional)

Optional Additions:

• White wine (for deglazing)

• Thyme or rosemary (for added herbaceous flavor)

• Spinach or arugula (for a touch of green)

Step-by-Step Instructions:

1. Sauté Mushrooms:

• In a large pan, heat olive oil over medium heat. Sauté the chopped onions until translucent, then add minced garlic and sliced mushrooms. Cook until mushrooms are golden brown.

2. Toast Barley:

• Add barley to the pan and toast for a couple of minutes until lightly golden, stirring occasionally.

3. Deglaze (Optional):

• For added depth of flavor, deglaze the pan with a splash of white wine, stirring to scrape up any flavorful bits from the bottom.

4. Simmer with Broth:

• Pour in vegetable broth gradually, one ladle at a time, stirring frequently. Allow the barley to absorb the liquid before adding more. Continue until the barley is cooked to your desired tenderness.

5. Finish with Parmesan:

• Stir in grated Parmesan cheese, allowing it to melt into the risotto and create a creamy texture.

6. Season to Taste:

• Season with salt and pepper to taste. Add fresh herbs like thyme or rosemary if desired.

7. Optional Greens:

• For added freshness, fold in spinach or arugula just before serving.

8. Garnish and Serve:

• Garnish with fresh parsley and additional Parmesan if desired. Serve hot.

Nutrition Information (Per Serving):

• Calories: 350 calories

• Protein: 12g

• Fat: 10g

• Carbohydrates: 55g

• Fiber: 10g

• Sugar: 3g

• Sodium: 700mg

FARRO SALAD WITH ROASTED VEGETABLES

Meal Description: The Farro Salad with Roasted Vegetables is a hearty and wholesome dish that combines the chewy texture of Farro with the robust flavors of roasted sweet potatoes and Brussels sprouts. Dried cranberries add a touch of sweetness, while a zesty vinaigrette ties all the elements together. This salad is a feast for the senses with its vibrant colors and a nutritious celebration of seasonal ingredients. Perfect for a light lunch or as a side dish, it's a delightful way to embrace the goodness of whole grains and vegetables.

Ingredients:

- 1 cup farro, cooked

- 2 cups sweet potatoes, peeled and cubed

- 2 cups Brussels sprouts, halved

- 1/2 cup dried cranberries

- Three tablespoons olive oil

- Salt and pepper to taste

For the Vinaigrette:

- Two tablespoons of balsamic vinegar

- One tablespoon of Dijon mustard

- One clove of garlic, minced

- 1/4 cup extra-virgin olive oil

- Salt and pepper to taste

Optional Additions:

- Toasted pecans or walnuts

- Feta or goat cheese crumbles

- Fresh herbs like parsley or thyme

Step-by-Step Instructions:

1. Roast Vegetables:

- Preheat the oven to 400°F (200°C).

- Toss cubed sweet potatoes and halved Brussels sprouts with olive oil, salt, and pepper.

- Roast in the oven until vegetables are golden brown and tender, approximately 25-30 minutes.

2. Cook Farro:

- Cook Farro according to package instructions. It should be tender but still have a pleasant chewiness.

3. Prepare Vinaigrette:

- Whisk together balsamic vinegar, Dijon mustard, minced garlic, extra-virgin olive oil, salt, and pepper in a small bowl.

4. Assemble the Salad:

- Combine cooked Farro, roasted sweet potatoes, Brussels sprouts, and dried cranberries in a large bowl.

5. Drizzle with Vinaigrette:

• Pour the vinaigrette over the salad. Toss gently to coat everything evenly.

6. Season to Taste:

• Adjust salt and pepper to taste.

7. Optional Additions:

• Sprinkle toasted pecans or walnuts over the salad for added crunch.

• Crumble feta or goat cheese for a creamy finish.

• Garnish with fresh herbs like parsley or thyme.

8. Serve and Enjoy:

• Serve the Farro Salad with Roasted Vegetables at room temperature or chilled.

Nutrition Information (Per Serving):

• Calories: 350 calories

• Protein: 8g

• Fat: 15g

• Carbohydrates: 50g

• Fiber: 8g

• Sugar: 10g

• Sodium: 150mg

QUINOA AND BLACK BEAN SALAD

Meal Description: The Quinoa and Black Bean Salad is a vibrant and refreshing dish that brings together protein-packed quinoa, fiber-rich black beans, sweet corn, crisp red onions, and the bright flavors of cilantro, all tied together with a zesty lime vinaigrette. This salad is a nutritional powerhouse and a burst of colors and textures, making it a perfect choice for a light lunch, a side dish, or a refreshing addition to your summer spread. It's a symphony of flavors that combines health and taste in every bite.

Ingredients:

• 1 cup quinoa, cooked

• One can (15 oz) black beans, drained and rinsed

• 1 cup corn kernels (fresh or frozen)

• 1/2 cup red onion, finely chopped

• 1/4 cup fresh cilantro, chopped

• Juice of 2 limes

For the Lime Vinaigrette:

• Three tablespoons olive oil

• Two tablespoons of lime juice

• One teaspoon of honey or maple syrup

• Salt and pepper to taste

Optional Additions:

• Diced tomatoes

• Avocado slices

• Jalapeño for a spicy kick

Step-by-Step Instructions:

1. Cook Quinoa:

• Prepare 1 cup of quinoa according to package instructions. Let it cool.

2. Prepare Vinaigrette:

• Whisk together olive oil, lime juice, honey or maple syrup, salt, and pepper in a small bowl to create the lime vinaigrette.

3. Combine Ingredients:

• Combine the cooked quinoa, black beans, corn, finely chopped red onion, and fresh cilantro in a large bowl.

4. Drizzle with Vinaigrette:

• Pour the lime vinaigrette over the quinoa and bean mixture. Toss gently to coat everything evenly.

5. Season to Taste:

• Adjust salt and pepper to taste.

6. Optional Additions:

• Add diced tomatoes, avocado slices, or jalapeño for additional flavors and textures if desired.

7. Chill (Optional):

• Allow the salad to chill in the refrigerator for about 15-30 minutes to enhance the flavors.

8. Serve and Enjoy:

• Serve the Quinoa and Black Bean Salad as a refreshing and nutritious dish.

Nutrition Information (Per Serving):

• Calories: 300 calories

• Protein: 10g

• Fat: 10g

• Carbohydrates: 45g

• Fiber: 8g

• Sugar: 3g

• Sodium: 350mg

BUCKWHEAT PANCAKES WITH BERRIES

Meal Description: Start your day on a wholesome note with Buckwheat Pancakes adorned with a medley of fresh berries and a dollop of creamy Greek Yogurt. These pancakes, made with nutty buckwheat flour and almond milk, offer a delightful combination of rich flavors and nutritional goodness. Topped with vibrant berries and a swirl of Greek Yogurt, this breakfast is a delicious way to incorporate whole grains, plant-based proteins, and antioxidants into your morning routine.

Ingredients:

For the Buckwheat Pancakes:

- 1 cup buckwheat flour

- 1 cup almond milk

- One tablespoon of maple syrup or honey

- One teaspoon of baking powder

- 1/2 teaspoon baking soda

- 1/4 teaspoon salt

- 1 tablespoon vegetable oil (for cooking)

For the Toppings:

• Mixed berries (strawberries, blueberries, raspberries)

• Greek Yogurt

Optional Additions:

• Chopped nuts (such as almonds or walnuts)

• Maple syrup for drizzling

• Shredded coconut for garnish

Step-by-Step Instructions:

1. Prepare the Buckwheat Pancake Batter:

• In a mixing bowl, whisk together buckwheat flour, almond milk, maple syrup or honey, baking powder, baking soda, and salt until you have a smooth batter.

2. Cook the Pancakes:

• Heat a griddle or non-stick pan over medium heat. Add a slight vegetable oil to coat the surface.

• Pour 1/4 cup portions of batter onto the griddle to form pancakes. Cook until bubbles appear on the surface, then flip and cook until golden brown on the other side.

3. Keep Warm:

• Place the cooked pancakes on a plate and keep warm.

4. Assemble the Pancakes:

• Stack the pancakes on individual plates.

5. Add Toppings:

• Top the pancakes with a generous amount of mixed berries.

6. Garnish with Greek Yogurt:

• Add a dollop of Greek Yogurt on top of the berries.

7. Optional Additions:

• Sprinkle chopped nuts, drizzle with maple syrup, and garnish with shredded coconut if desired.

8. Serve and Enjoy:

• Serve the Buckwheat Pancakes with Berries immediately while warm.

Nutrition Information (Per Serving):

• Calories: 250 calories

• Protein: 8g

• Fat: 8g

• Carbohydrates: 38g

• Fiber: 6g

• Sugar: 8g

• Sodium: 400mg

MILLET AND VEGETABLE STIR-FRY

Meal Description: Embrace a wholesome and plant-based delight with Millet and Vegetable Stir-Fry. Nutty millet forms the base of this dish, complemented by a colorful array of broccoli, carrots, snap peas, and protein-rich tofu. The entire stir-fry is infused with the savory flavors of soy sauce, creating a balanced and satisfying meal that's delicious and packed with essential nutrients. Enjoy the goodness of whole grains and a variety of vegetables in every flavorful bite.

Ingredients:

For the Millet and Vegetable Stir-Fry:

- 1 cup millet, cooked

- 1 cup broccoli florets

- 1 cup carrots, julienned

- 1 cup snap peas, ends trimmed

- 1 cup firm tofu, cubed

- Two tablespoons of soy sauce

- One tablespoon of vegetable oil

- One clove of garlic, minced

- One teaspoon of ginger, grated

- Sesame seeds for garnish (optional)

- Green onions, sliced for garnish (optional)

Optional Additions:

- Red bell pepper strips

- Water chestnuts

- Baby corn

- Sriracha or chili garlic sauce (for added heat)

Step-by-Step Instructions:

1. Cook Millet:

- Prepare 1 cup of cooked millet according to package instructions. Fluff with a fork and set aside.

2. Sauté Tofu:

- In a large wok or pan, heat vegetable oil over medium-high heat. Add cubed tofu and sauté until golden brown on all sides.

3. Add Vegetables:

- Add minced garlic and grated ginger to the pan. Stir in broccoli, carrots, and snap peas. Sauté until the vegetables are crisp-tender.

4. Combine with Millet:

- Add the cooked millet to the pan with the vegetables and tofu. Mix well to combine.

5. Drizzle with Soy Sauce:

- Pour soy sauce over the stir-fry and toss to coat the ingredients evenly.

6. Optional Additions:

• Toss in red bell pepper strips, water chestnuts, or baby corn for added color and flavor.

7. Season to Taste:

• Adjust the seasoning with additional soy sauce if needed. Add Sriracha or chili garlic sauce for extra heat if desired.

8. Garnish and Serve:

• Garnish with sesame seeds and sliced green onions. Serve the Millet and Vegetable Stir-Fry hot.

Nutrition Information (Per Serving):

• Calories: 350 calories

• Protein: 12g

• Fat: 10g

• Carbohydrates: 50g

• Fiber: 8g

• Sugar: 3g

• Sodium: 600mg

OATMEAL WITH FRESH FRUIT

Meal Description: Start your day with a bowl of wholesome Oatmeal with Fresh Fruit, a nutritious and satisfying breakfast that combines the heartiness of rolled oats with the sweetness of ripe banana and a burst of vibrant berries. Almond milk adds a creamy texture, while chia seeds contribute a dose of omega-3 fatty acids and additional texture. This delightful bowl is rich in fiber and essential nutrients and a delicious way to kick off your morning with a burst of energy.

Ingredients:

For the Oatmeal:

- 1/2 cup rolled oats

- 1 cup almond milk (or any milk of choice)

- One ripe banana, sliced

- Mixed berries (strawberries, blueberries, raspberries)

- One tablespoon of chia seeds

Optional Additions:

- Honey or maple syrup for sweetness

- Nuts (such as almonds or walnuts) for crunch

- A sprinkle of cinnamon or nutmeg for extra flavor

Step-by-Step Instructions:

1. Cook Oatmeal:

• In a saucepan, combine rolled oats and almond milk. Cook over medium heat, stirring occasionally, until the oats are creamy and tender.

2. Add Banana Slices:

• Stir in sliced banana to infuse natural sweetness into the Oatmeal.

3. Prepare Berries:

• Wash and prepare a mix of berries (strawberries, blueberries, raspberries).

4. Assemble the Bowl:

• Once the Oatmeal is cooked to your desired consistency, transfer it to a serving bowl.

5. Top with Fresh Fruit:

• Arrange the mixed berries on top of the Oatmeal.

6. Sprinkle with Chia Seeds:

• Sprinkle chia seeds over the fresh fruit for added texture and nutritional benefits.

7. Optional Additions:

• Drizzle with honey or maple syrup for additional sweetness if desired.

• Add a handful of nuts for a delightful crunch.

• Sprinkle a pinch of cinnamon or nutmeg for extra flavor.

8. Serve and Enjoy:

• Serve the Oatmeal with Fresh Fruit and enjoy a nourishing breakfast bowl.

Nutrition Information (Per Serving):

- Calories: 300 calories
- Protein: 8g
- Fat: 10g
- Carbohydrates: 50g
- Fiber: 10g
- Sugar: 15g
- Sodium: 150mg

WHOLE WHEAT WRAP WITH HUMMUS AND VEGGIES

Meal Description: Elevate your lunchtime with a Whole Wheat Wrap filled with creamy hummus and a medley of fresh, crisp vegetables. This quick and healthy wrap is not only delicious but also a balanced combination of whole grains, protein-packed hummus, and a variety of colorful veggies. The full wheat wrap serves as a nutritious vessel for this plant-based delight, making it a satisfying and convenient meal that's perfect for a busy day.

Ingredients:

For the Whole Wheat Wrap:

• One whole wheat wrap

• Two tablespoons hummus (store-bought or homemade)

Vegetable Fillings:

• Cucumber, thinly sliced

• Tomatoes, sliced

• Fresh spinach leaves

Optional Additions:

• Red onion, thinly sliced

• Bell peppers, thinly sliced

• Avocado slices

• Sprouts for added crunch

Step-by-Step Instructions:

1. Prep the Whole Wheat Wrap:

• Lay the whole wheat wrap on a clean surface.

2. Spread Hummus:

• Spread a generous layer of hummus evenly over the surface of the wrap.

3. Add Vegetables:

• Layer on the sliced cucumber, tomatoes, and fresh spinach leaves.

4. Optional Additions:

• Add thinly sliced red onion, bell peppers, avocado slices, or sprouts for extra flavor and texture if desired.

5. Fold and Roll:

• Carefully fold the sides of the wrap and then roll it from the bottom to create a tight, compact wrap.

6. Slice (Optional):

• You can slice the wrap in half diagonally or into smaller portions for easier handling.

7. Serve and Enjoy:

• Serve the Whole Wheat Wrap with Hummus and Veggies immediately and savor a quick, nutritious, and delicious meal.

Nutrition Information (Per Serving):

- Calories: 300 calories
- Protein: 10g
- Fat: 12g
- Carbohydrates: 40g
- Fiber: 8g
- Sugar: 3g
- Sodium: 500mg

CHAPTER FIVE

Lean Proteins Recipes

Baked Salmon with Lemon and Dill

Meal Description: Elevate your dinner with a light, flavorful Baked Salmon with Lemon and Dill. This simple yet elegant dish features succulent salmon fillets infused with the zesty brightness of lemon and the aromatic freshness of dill. Baked to perfection with a drizzle of olive oil, this seafood delight is delicious and a healthy source of omega-3 fatty acids. Enjoy the delicate balance of citrus and herbs in every forkful of this nourishing and easy-to-prepare meal.

Ingredients:

- Salmon fillets (as many as needed)

- One lemon, thinly sliced

- Fresh dill, chopped

- Two tablespoons of olive oil

- Salt and pepper to taste

Optional Additions:

- Garlic cloves, minced

- Paprika for a touch of warmth

Step-by-Step Instructions:

1. Preheat the Oven:

- Preheat your Oven to 375°F (190°C).

2. Prepare Salmon Fillets:

- Pat the salmon fillets dry with a paper towel. Place them on a baking sheet lined with parchment paper or lightly greased.

3. Season with Olive Oil, Salt, and Pepper:

• Drizzle olive oil over the salmon fillets, ensuring they are evenly coated. Season with salt and pepper to taste.

4. Add Lemon Slices:

• Lay thin slices of lemon over the salmon fillets. This imparts flavor and helps keep the salmon moist during baking.

5. Sprinkle with Dill:

• Sprinkle chopped fresh dill over the salmon, covering it evenly for that delightful herbal aroma.

6. Optional Additions:

• If desired, add minced garlic cloves or a sprinkle of paprika for extra depth of flavor.

7. Bake in the Oven:

• Place the baking sheet in the preheated Oven and bake for approximately 15-20 minutes or until the salmon is cooked through and flakes easily with a fork.

8. Broil for Crispy Top (Optional):

• For a slightly crispy top, you can switch the Oven to broil for the last 2-3 minutes of baking. Keep a close eye to prevent burning.

9. Serve and Enjoy:

• Carefully transfer the baked salmon with lemon and dill to serving plates. Serve immediately.

Nutrition Information (Per Serving):

• Calories: 300 calories

• Protein: 25g

- Fat: 20g
- Carbohydrates: 2g
- Fiber: 1g
- Sugar: 0g
- Sodium: 80mg

GRILLED CHICKEN SALAD

Meal Description: Indulge in a light and flavorful Grilled Chicken Salad that brings together the succulence of grilled chicken breast, the freshness of mixed greens, sweet bursts of cherry tomatoes, and the tangy richness of balsamic vinaigrette. This salad is a feast for the senses with its vibrant colors and a wholesome and satisfying meal that strikes the perfect balance between protein and greens. Enjoy the simplicity and deliciousness of this grilled chicken salad for a quick and nutritious lunch or dinner.

Ingredients:

• Grilled chicken breast, sliced

• Mixed greens (lettuce, spinach, arugula)

• Cherry tomatoes, halved

• Balsamic vinaigrette dressing

Optional Additions:

• Cucumbers, sliced

• Red onion, thinly sliced

• Avocado slices

• Crumbled feta or goat cheese

• Toasted nuts (such as almonds or walnuts)

Step-by-Step Instructions:

1. Grill Chicken Breast:

• Grill the chicken breast until fully cooked. Allow it to rest for a few minutes before slicing it into thin strips.

2. Prepare Salad Greens:

• Combine mixed greens, cherry tomatoes, and any additional salad ingredients you prefer in a large bowl.

3. Add Grilled Chicken:

• Place the sliced grilled chicken on top of the salad greens.

4. Drizzle with Balsamic Vinaigrette:

• Drizzle balsamic vinaigrette over the salad. Start with a small amount and add more according to your taste preference.

5. Toss Gently:

• Gently toss the salad to ensure that the grilled chicken and dressing are evenly distributed.

6. Optional Garnishes:

• Garnish the salad with additional ingredients like sliced cucumbers, red onions, avocado slices, crumbled feta or goat cheese, and toasted nuts if desired.

7. Serve and Enjoy:

• Serve the Grilled Chicken Salad immediately, savoring the combination of tender chicken, crisp greens, and the delightful balsamic vinaigrette.

Nutrition Information (Per Serving):

• Calories: 350 calories

- Protein: 30g
- Fat: 15g
- Carbohydrates: 20g
- Fiber: 5g
- Sugar: 8g
- Sodium: 500mg

TOFU AND VEGETABLE SKEWERS

Meal Description: Immerse yourself in the delightful world of plant-based cuisine with Tofu and Vegetable Skewers. These skewers feature marinated tofu cubes paired with vibrant bell peppers, juicy cherry tomatoes, and tender zucchini, all grilled to perfection. The finishing touch comes from a savory teriyaki marinade that adds a burst of flavor to this colorful and satisfying dish. Whether enjoyed as a main course or a delightful appetizer, these skewers are a celebration of fresh, wholesome ingredients and bold flavors.

Ingredients:

• Firm Tofu, cubed

• Bell peppers (assorted colors), cut into chunks

• Cherry tomatoes

• Zucchini, sliced

• Teriyaki marinade

Optional Additions:

• Red onion, cut into wedges

• Pineapple chunks for a sweet twist

• Sesame seeds for garnish

• Fresh cilantro for garnish

Step-by-Step Instructions:

1. Prepare Tofu:

• Press the Tofu to remove excess water, then cut it into bite-sized cubes.

2. Marinate Tofu:

• Place the tofu cubes in a bowl and marinate them in teriyaki marinade. Allow them to soak up the flavors for at least 30 minutes.

3. Prepare Vegetables:

• Cut bell peppers into chunks, slice zucchini, and gather cherry tomatoes. If using, cut red onion into wedges.

4. Assemble Skewers:

• Thread the marinated tofu cubes and assorted vegetables onto skewers, alternating for a colorful presentation.

5. Grill or Bake:

• Grill the skewers on an outdoor grill or indoor grill pan, turning occasionally, until the vegetables are tender and the Tofu is lightly browned. Alternatively, you can bake them in the Oven.

6. Baste with Marinade:

• While grilling, baste the skewers with additional teriyaki marinade for added flavor.

7. Optional Garnishes:

• Garnish with sesame seeds and fresh cilantro for an extra burst of flavor.

8. Serve and Enjoy:

• Serve the Tofu and Vegetable Skewers hot as a standalone dish or paired with rice or a side of your choice.

Nutrition Information (Per Serving):

• Calories: 250 calories

• Protein: 15g

• Fat: 10g

• Carbohydrates: 25g

• Fiber: 5g

• Sugar: 10g

• Sodium: 600mg

TURKEY AND QUINOA STUFFED PEPPERS

Meal Description: Savor the goodness of lean ground turkey and protein-rich quinoa in this delightful Turkey and Quinoa Stuffed Peppers recipe. These peppers are generously filled with a flavorful mixture of ground turkey, quinoa, black beans, tomatoes, and a blend of aromatic spices. Baked to perfection, this dish offers a burst of savory flavors and a well-balanced combination of essential nutrients. Enjoy a wholesome and satisfying meal with these stuffed peppers that are as nourishing as they are delicious.

Ingredients:

• Bell peppers (assorted colors), halved and seeds removed

• Ground turkey

• Quinoa, cooked

• Black beans, canned and drained

• Diced tomatoes (fresh or canned)

• Spices (cumin, chili powder, paprika, garlic powder, salt, and pepper)

Optional Additions:

- Shredded cheese for topping

- Fresh cilantro or parsley for garnish

- Avocado slices or guacamole on the side

Step-by-Step Instructions:

1. Prepare Bell Peppers:

- Cut bell peppers in half lengthwise, removing seeds and membranes. Parboil the peppers in boiling water for 2-3 minutes to soften slightly. Drain and set aside.

2. Cook Quinoa:

- Cook quinoa according to package instructions. Set aside.

3. Cook Ground Turkey:

- In a skillet over medium heat, cook ground turkey until browned and cooked through. Drain any excess fat.

4. Combine Ingredients:

- In a large bowl, combine cooked ground turkey, cooked quinoa, black beans, diced tomatoes, and spices (cumin, chili powder, paprika, garlic powder, salt, and pepper). Mix well to create a flavorful filling.

5. Preheat Oven:

- Preheat your Oven to 375°F (190°C).

6. Fill Peppers:

- Stuff each bell pepper half with the turkey and quinoa mixture, pressing down gently to pack the filling.

7. Bake:

- Place the stuffed peppers in a baking dish. Bake in the preheated Oven for 25-30 minutes or until the peppers are tender.

8. Optional Cheese Topping:

• If desired, sprinkle shredded cheese on top of the stuffed peppers during the last 5 minutes of baking.

9. Garnish and Serve:

• Garnish with fresh cilantro or parsley. Serve the Turkey and Quinoa Stuffed Peppers hot, with avocado slices or guacamole on the side if desired.

Nutrition Information (Per Serving):

• Calories: 300 calories

• Protein: 25g

• Fat: 10g

• Carbohydrates: 30g

• Fiber: 8g

• Sugar: 5g

• Sodium: 600mg

LENTIL AND VEGETABLE SOUP

Meal Description: Warm your soul with a bowl of hearty lentils and vegetable soup. This nourishing soup brings together the wholesome goodness of lentils, the crunch of carrots and celery, and the richness of tomatoes, all in a flavorful vegetable broth. This simple yet satisfying dish is a celebration of plant-based ingredients that provide comfort and a healthy dose of fiber and essential nutrients. Perfect for chilly days or whenever you crave a comforting and nutritious meal.

Ingredients:

• Lentils (green or brown), rinsed and drained

• Carrots, diced

• Celery, diced

• Tomatoes, diced

• Vegetable broth

• Olive oil

• Onion, finely chopped

• Garlic, minced

• Spices (cumin, paprika, thyme, bay leaves)

• Salt and pepper to taste

Optional Additions:

• Spinach or kale for added greens

• Lemon juice for a touch of acidity

• Fresh parsley for garnish

• Crusty bread for serving

Step-by-Step Instructions:

1. Sauté Onion and Garlic:

• In a large pot, heat olive oil over medium heat. Add finely chopped onion and minced garlic. Sauté until the onion is translucent.

2. Add Vegetables:

• Add diced carrots and celery to the pot. Cook for a few minutes until the vegetables start to soften.

3. Add Lentils and Tomatoes:

• Add rinsed and drained lentils, diced tomatoes, and any optional greens (spinach or kale) to the pot. Stir to combine.

4. Season with Spices:

• Season the soup with cumin, paprika, thyme, bay leaves, salt, and pepper. Adjust the seasoning according to your taste preference.

5. Pour in Vegetable Broth:

• Pour vegetable broth into the pot, ensuring that the lentils and vegetables are well-covered. Bring the soup to a gentle boil.

6. Simmer:

• Reduce the heat to low, cover the pot, and let the

soup simmer for 20-25 minutes or until the lentils and vegetables are tender.

7. Optional Lemon Juice:

• If desired, add a squeeze of lemon juice for a touch of acidity. Adjust the seasoning as needed.

8. Serve and Garnish:

• Ladle the Lentil and Vegetable Soup into bowls. Garnish with fresh parsley and serve hot. Pair with crusty bread for a complete and satisfying meal.

Nutrition Information (Per Serving):

• Calories: 250 calories

• Protein: 15g

• Fat: 3g

• Carbohydrates: 45g

• Fiber: 15g

• Sugar: 8g

• Sodium: 800mg

SHRIMP AND QUINOA STIR-FRY

Meal Description: Elevate your dinner with the vibrant and nutritious Shrimp and Quinoa Stir-Fry. This quick and flavorful dish combines succulent shrimp, protein-packed quinoa, and a medley of crisp broccoli and snap peas, all coated in a savory soy sauce. This stir-fry not only delights your taste buds with its fresh ingredients but also provides a well-balanced meal that's rich in both flavor and nutrients. Enjoy the simplicity and goodness of this delightful shrimp and quinoa creation.

Ingredients:

• Shrimp, peeled and deveined

• Quinoa, cooked

• Broccoli florets

• Snap peas, ends trimmed

• Soy sauce

• Sesame oil

• Garlic, minced

• Ginger, grated

• Green onions, sliced for garnish

Optional Additions:

• Carrots, julienned

• Bell peppers, sliced

• Red chili flakes for heat

• Sesame seeds for garnish

Step-by-Step Instructions:

1. Cook Quinoa:

• Cook quinoa according to package instructions. Set aside.

2. Prep Shrimp and Vegetables:

• In a wok or large skillet, heat sesame oil over medium-high heat. Add minced garlic and grated ginger, sautéing until fragrant.

3. Stir-Fry Shrimp:

• Add shrimp to the wok and stir-fry until they turn pink and opaque. Remove shrimp from the wok and set aside.

4. Cook Vegetables:

• In the same wok, add a bit more sesame oil if needed. Add broccoli florets and snap peas, stir-frying until they are tender-crisp.

5. Combine Shrimp and Quinoa:

• Return the cooked shrimp to the wok, along with the cooked quinoa. Toss everything together to combine.

6. Pour Soy Sauce:

• Pour soy sauce over the stir-fry, ensuring an even coating. Adjust the amount to your taste preference.

7. Optional Additions:

• Add julienned carrots or sliced bell peppers for

additional color and flavor if desired. For heat, sprinkle red chili flakes.

8. Garnish and Serve:

• Garnish the Shrimp and Quinoa Stir-Fry with sliced green onions and sesame seeds. Serve hot.

Nutrition Information (Per Serving):

• Calories: 350 calories

• Protein: 25g

• Fat: 8g

• Carbohydrates: 45g

• Fiber: 6g

• Sugar: 3g

• Sodium: 800mg

BAKED COD
WITH HERBS

Meal Description: Experience the light and fresh flavors of the ocean with Baked Cod with Herbs. This simple and elegant dish features tender cod fillets seasoned with garlic, thyme, and a splash of lemon, all baked to perfection with a drizzle of olive oil. The result is a mouthwatering creation that showcases the delicate taste of cod and brings a burst of aromatic herbs to the forefront. This easy-to-make Baked Cod with Herbs offers a wholesome and delightful seafood experience.

Ingredients:

• Cod fillets

• Garlic, minced

• Fresh thyme leaves

• Lemon, thinly sliced

• Olive oil

• Salt and pepper to taste

Optional Additions:

• Cherry tomatoes for a burst of freshness

• Capers for added tanginess

• Parsley for garnish

Step-by-Step Instructions:

1. Preheat the Oven:

• Preheat your Oven to 375°F (190°C).

2. Prepare Cod Fillets:

• Pat the cod fillets dry with a paper towel and place them on a baking sheet lined with parchment paper or lightly greased.

3. Season with Garlic and Thyme:

• Spread minced garlic and fresh thyme leaves evenly over the cod fillets.

4. Drizzle with Olive Oil:

• Drizzle olive oil over the cod fillets, ensuring they are lightly coated. This adds moisture and enhances the flavors.

5. Arrange Lemon Slices:

• Place thin slices of lemon on top of the cod fillets for a citrusy kick.

6. Season with Salt and Pepper:

• Season the cod fillets with salt and pepper to taste.

7. Optional Additions:

• Scatter cherry tomatoes around the cod fillets or sprinkle capers for added flavor if desired.

8. Bake in the Oven:

• Bake the cod in the preheated Oven for approximately 15-20 minutes or until the fish is opaque and easily flakes with a fork.

9. Broil for Crispy Top (Optional):

• For a slightly crispy top, you can switch the Oven to broil for the last 2-3 minutes of baking. Keep a close eye to prevent burning.

10. Garnish and Serve:

• Garnish the Baked Cod with Herbs with fresh parsley if desired. Serve hot.

Nutrition Information (Per Serving):

• Calories: 200 calories

• Protein: 25g

• Fat: 8g

• Carbohydrates: 2g

• Fiber: 1g

• Sugar: 0g

• Sodium: 400mg

CHICKPEA SALAD WITH FETA

Meal Description: Savor the vibrant flavors of the Mediterranean with Chickpea Salad with Feta. This refreshing salad brings together protein-packed chickpeas, crisp cucumber, juicy cherry tomatoes, and the creamy goodness of feta cheese—all tossed in a light and flavorful olive oil dressing. Whether enjoyed as a satisfying side dish or a light main course, this salad is a celebration of fresh ingredients that harmonize beautifully to create a delightful and nutritious culinary experience.

Ingredients:

• Chickpeas (canned or cooked), drained and rinsed

• Cucumber, diced

• Cherry tomatoes, halved

• Feta cheese, crumbled

• Olive oil

• Salt and pepper to taste

Optional Additions:

• Red onion, finely chopped

• Kalamata olives for a briny kick

• Fresh parsley or mint for garnish

• Lemon juice for extra brightness

Step-by-Step Instructions:

1. Prepare Chickpeas:

• If using canned chickpeas, drain and rinse them thoroughly. If using dried chickpeas, cook them according to package instructions and let them cool.

2. Combine Ingredients:

• Combine chickpeas, diced cucumber, halved cherry tomatoes, and crumbled feta cheese in a large bowl.

3. Drizzle with Olive Oil:

• Drizzle olive oil over the salad ingredients. Toss gently to coat everything evenly.

4. Season with Salt and Pepper:

• Season the Chickpea Salad with Feta with salt and pepper to taste. Adjust the seasoning as needed.

5. Optional Additions:

• Add finely chopped red onion, Kalamata olives, or a squeeze of lemon juice for extra flavor.

6. Toss Gently:

• Gently toss the salad to ensure the ingredients are well combined and coated with the olive oil dressing.

7. Garnish and Serve:

• Garnish the Chickpea Salad with Feta with fresh parsley or mint if desired. Serve immediately or refrigerate until ready to serve.

Nutrition Information (Per Serving):

- Calories: 300 calories
- Protein: 15g
- Fat: 15g
- Carbohydrates: 30g
- Fiber: 8g
- Sugar: 5g
- Sodium: 600mg

GREEK YOGURT CHICKEN WRAP

Meal Description: Indulge in a healthy and delicious meal with the Greek Yogurt Chicken Wrap. This wrap combines tender grilled chicken strips with the creamy goodness of Greek yogurt, crisp cucumber, and juicy tomatoes—all wrapped in a wholesome whole wheat wrap. The result is a protein-packed delight that satisfies your taste buds and provides a balanced and nutritious meal. Enjoy this flavorful and convenient wrap for a quick lunch or a light dinner.

Ingredients:

- Grilled chicken strips

- Greek yogurt

- Cucumber, thinly sliced

- Tomatoes, sliced

- Whole wheat wrap

Optional Additions:

- Red onion, thinly sliced

- Kalamata olives for a Mediterranean touch

- Fresh spinach leaves for added greens

- Feta cheese crumbles for extra richness

Step-by-Step Instructions:

1. Prepare Ingredients:

• Ensure that the grilled chicken strips, Greek yogurt, cucumber, and tomatoes are ready for assembly.

2. Warm the Whole Wheat Wrap:

• Warm the whole wheat wrap for a few seconds in a microwave or on a skillet to make it more pliable.

3. Assemble the Wrap:

• Lay the whole wheat wrap on a flat surface. Place a layer of Greek yogurt in the center of the wrap.

4. Add Grilled Chicken Strips:

• Arrange grilled chicken strips on top of the Greek yogurt, creating an even layer.

5. Layer with Vegetables:

• Add thinly sliced cucumber and tomato slices on top of the chicken. If desired, include additional ingredients like red onion, Kalamata olives, fresh spinach leaves, or feta cheese crumbles.

6. Fold and Roll:

• Carefully fold the sides of the whole wheat wrap over the fillings and then roll it tightly from the bottom, creating a wrap.

7. Serve and Enjoy:

• Slice the Greek Yogurt Chicken Wrap diagonally and serve immediately. Alternatively, wrap it in parchment paper for a convenient on-the-go meal.

Nutrition Information (Per Serving):

• Calories: 400 calories

- Protein: 30g
- Fat: 15g
- Carbohydrates: 35g
- Fiber: 8g
- Sugar: 5g
- Sodium: 600mg

BLACK BEAN AND VEGETABLE QUESADILLA

Meal Description: Embark on a culinary journey with the Black Bean and Vegetable Quesadilla—a delightful fusion of black beans, colorful bell peppers, onions, and gooey cheese, all nestled within a whole wheat tortilla. This savory and satisfying dish celebrates the richness of plant-based ingredients and offers a perfect balance of flavors and textures. Enjoy this quesadilla as a hearty lunch or a quick dinner, bringing a burst of taste to your plate in every bite.

Ingredients:

- Black beans, canned and drained
- Bell peppers (assorted colors), thinly sliced
- Onion, thinly sliced
- Whole wheat tortilla
- Cheese (cheddar, Monterey Jack, or a blend), shredded
- Olive oil for cooking

Optional Additions:

- Avocado slices or guacamole for creaminess

• Salsa or pico de gallo for a tangy kick

• Sour cream or Greek yogurt for dipping

• Fresh cilantro or green onions for garnish

Step-by-Step Instructions:

1. Prep Vegetables and Beans:

• Thinly slice bell peppers and onions. Ensure that the black beans are drained and ready to use.

2. Cook Vegetables:

• In a skillet over medium heat, add a bit of olive oil. Sauté the sliced bell peppers and onions until they are tender-crisp. Add black beans to the mixture and heat through.

3. Assemble Quesadilla:

• Place a whole wheat tortilla on a flat surface. Layer the sautéed vegetable and black bean mixture on one half of the tortilla.

4. Add Cheese:

• Sprinkle a generous amount of shredded cheese over the vegetable and black bean mixture.

5. Fold and Cook:

• Fold the tortilla in half, covering the vegetable and bean filling. In the same skillet, cook the quesadilla over medium heat until the cheese is melted and the tortilla is golden brown on both sides.

6. Optional Additions:

• If desired, top the cooked quesadilla with avocado slices or guacamole, salsa or pico de gallo, and a dollop of sour cream or Greek yogurt. Garnish with fresh cilantro or green onions.

7. Slice and Serve:

• Slice the Black Bean and Vegetable Quesadilla into wedges and serve hot.

Nutrition Information (Per Serving):

• Calories: 350 calories

• Protein: 15g

• Fat: 15g

• Carbohydrates: 40g

• Fiber: 8g

• Sugar: 3g

• Sodium: 600mg

CHAPTER SIX

Healthy Fats Recipes

Avocado and Tomato Toast

Meal Description: Elevate your brunch experience with the Avocado and Tomato Toast—a classic and wholesome combination that brings together the creamy richness of Avocado, the juiciness of cherry tomatoes, and the nutty flavor of whole grain bread. Drizzled with a touch of olive oil, this toast is a visual delight and a nutritious treat that's quick to prepare. Enjoy the simplicity and freshness of this toast for a delightful start to your day.

Ingredients:

• Whole grain bread slices

• Avocado, ripe and sliced

• Cherry tomatoes, halved

• Olive oil

• Salt and pepper to taste

Optional Additions:

• Red pepper flakes for a hint of spice

• Lemon juice for extra brightness

• Fresh basil or cilantro for garnish

• Feta cheese crumbles for added richness

Step-by-Step Instructions:

1. Toast the Bread:

• Toast whole-grain bread slices until they reach your desired level of crispiness.

2. Prepare Avocado:

• While the bread is toasting, slice a ripe avocado and fan the slices for easy placement on the toast.

3. Assemble the Toast:

• Place the toasted whole-grain bread on a plate. Arrange the sliced Avocado on top of the toast.

4. Add Cherry Tomatoes:

• Halve cherry tomatoes and distribute them evenly over the avocado slices.

5. Drizzle with Olive Oil:

• Drizzle a small amount of olive oil over the avocado and tomato topping. This adds a touch of richness and enhances the flavors.

6. Season with Salt and Pepper:

• Season the Avocado and Tomato Toast with salt and pepper to taste. Adjust the Seasoning according to your preference.

7. Optional Additions:

• If desired, sprinkle red pepper flakes for a hint of spice, squeeze fresh lemon juice for extra brightness, garnish with fresh basil or cilantro, or add feta cheese crumbles for added richness.

8. Serve and Enjoy:

• Serve the Avocado and Tomato Toast immediately while the bread is still warm.

Nutrition Information (Per Serving):

• Calories: 250 calories

• Protein: 8g

• Fat: 15g

- Carbohydrates: 25g
- Fiber: 8g
- Sugar: 3g
- Sodium: 300mg

SALMON AND AVOCADO SALAD

Meal Description: Elevate your salad experience with the Salmon and Avocado Salad—a delightful ensemble of mixed greens, succulent smoked salmon, creamy Avocado, and a zesty lemon vinaigrette. This salad offers a burst of fresh and vibrant flavors and a rich source of omega-3 fatty acids, proteins, and essential nutrients. Enjoy the balance of textures and the nourishing goodness of this salmon and avocado creation for a light and satisfying meal.

Ingredients:

• Mixed greens (lettuce, spinach, arugula, etc.)

• Smoked salmon slices

• Avocado, sliced

• Lemon vinaigrette

Lemon Vinaigrette:

• Olive oil

• Lemon juice

• Dijon mustard

• Honey or maple syrup (optional)

• Salt and pepper to taste

Optional Additions:

- Cherry tomatoes for sweetness

- Cucumber slices for freshness

- Red onion, thinly sliced

- Capers for a briny kick

- Toasted pine nuts for crunch

Step-by-Step Instructions:

1. Prepare Lemon Vinaigrette:

- Whisk together olive oil, lemon juice, Dijon mustard, honey or maple syrup (if using), salt, and pepper in a small bowl. Adjust the sweetness and acidity to your taste.

2. Assemble the Salad:

- Combine mixed greens, smoked salmon slices, and sliced Avocado in a large bowl.

3. Drizzle with Lemon Vinaigrette:

- Drizzle the prepared lemon vinaigrette over the salad. Toss gently to coat the ingredients evenly.

4. Optional Additions:

- Add cherry tomatoes, cucumber slices, thinly sliced red onion, capers, or toasted pine nuts for additional flavors and textures if desired.

5. Serve Immediately:

- Serve the Salmon and Avocado Salad immediately to enjoy the freshness and vibrant flavors.

Nutrition Information (Per Serving):

- Calories: 400 calories

- Protein: 20g
- Fat: 30g
- Carbohydrates: 15g
- Fiber: 8g
- Sugar: 5g
- Sodium: 600mg

ALMOND-CRUSTED TILAPIA

Meal Description: Experience a burst of flavor with Almond-Crusted Tilapia—a delightful combination of tender tilapia fillets coated in crunchy almonds and enhanced with the zesty freshness of lemon zest. This dish offers a satisfying crunch and a rich source of omega-3 fatty acids and essential nutrients. With a drizzle of olive oil for added richness, this almond-crusted tilapia is a perfect blend of textures and tastes that's quick to prepare and delightful to savor.

Ingredients:

• Tilapia fillets

• Almonds, finely chopped or ground

• Lemon zest

• Olive oil

Optional Additions:

• Fresh parsley, chopped, for garnish

• Garlic powder for extra flavor

• Salt and pepper to taste

Step-by-Step Instructions:

1. Preheat the Oven:

• Preheat your Oven to 400°F (200°C).

2. Prepare Almond Coating:

• Finely chop or grind almonds to create a coarse texture. Mix in lemon zest, garlic powder (if using), salt, and pepper.

3. Coat Tilapia Fillets:

• Pat the tilapia fillets dry with a paper towel. Dip each fillet into the almond mixture, pressing the coating onto the fish to ensure it adheres.

4. Place on Baking Sheet:

• Place the almond-crusted tilapia fillets on a baking sheet lined with parchment paper or lightly greased.

5. Drizzle with Olive Oil:

• Drizzle a small amount of olive oil over the top of each fillet. This helps to enhance the flavor and promotes a crispy texture.

6. Bake in the Oven:

• Bake the almond-crusted tilapia in the preheated Oven for approximately 12-15 minutes or until the fish is cooked through and the coating is golden brown.

7. Optional Broiling:

• If you desire a crispier top, you can switch the Oven to broil for the last 2-3 minutes, keeping a close eye to prevent burning.

8. Garnish and Serve:

• Garnish the Almond-Crusted Tilapia with fresh chopped parsley. Serve hot.

Nutrition Information (Per Serving):

- Calories: 250 calories
- Protein: 25g
- Fat: 15g
- Carbohydrates: 5g
- Fiber: 3g
- Sugar: 1g
- Sodium: 400mg

WALNUT AND BLUEBERRY QUINOA BOWL

Meal Description: Start your day on a wholesome note with the Walnut and Blueberry Quinoa Bowl —a nourishing blend of protein-rich quinoa, crunchy walnuts, juicy blueberries, and a touch of sweetness from honey. This vibrant bowl provides a satisfying crunch and a powerhouse of nutrients, including antioxidants, omega-3 fatty acids, and essential vitamins. Enjoy this delightful quinoa bowl as a fulfilling breakfast or a nutritious snack that fuels your body and delights your taste buds.

Ingredients:

• Quinoa, cooked

• Walnuts, chopped

• Blueberries

• Honey

Optional Additions:

• Greek yogurt for creaminess

• Chia seeds for extra fiber

• Cinnamon for a warm flavor

• Mint leaves for garnish

Step-by-Step Instructions:

1. Cook Quinoa:

• Cook quinoa according to package instructions. Fluff the cooked quinoa with a fork.

2. Assemble the Bowl:

• In a bowl, place a serving of cooked quinoa as the base.

3. Add Walnuts:

• Sprinkle chopped walnuts over the quinoa, distributing them evenly.

4. Top with Blueberries:

• Add a generous handful of fresh blueberries to the bowl. The vibrant color adds both visual appeal and natural sweetness.

5. Drizzle with Honey:

• Drizzle honey over the Walnut and Blueberry Quinoa Bowl to add a touch of sweetness. Adjust the amount to your liking.

6. Optional Additions:

• If desired, add a dollop of Greek yogurt for creaminess, sprinkle chia seeds for extra fiber, or dust the bowl with a pinch of cinnamon for a warm flavor.

7. Garnish and Serve:

• Garnish the bowl with fresh mint leaves for a burst of freshness. Serve and enjoy.

Nutrition Information (Per Serving):

- Calories: 350 calories
- Protein: 10g
- Fat: 15g
- Carbohydrates: 45g
- Fiber: 8g
- Sugar: 15g
- Sodium: 20mg

OLIVE TAPENADE

Recipe Description: Transport yourself to the Mediterranean with Olive Tapenade—a savory and briny spread made with Kalamata olives, capers, garlic, and olive oil. This versatile dish serves as a delightful appetizer or snack, perfect for spreading on whole-grain crackers. The combination of bold flavors and rich textures makes Olive Tapenade an excellent addition to your culinary repertoire, whether you're hosting a gathering or simply looking for a flavorful treat.

Ingredients:

• Kalamata olives, pitted

• Capers drained

• Garlic cloves, minced

• Olive oil

• Whole grain crackers for serving

Optional Additions:

• Fresh parsley, chopped, for garnish

• Lemon zest for a citrusy kick

• Sundried tomatoes for sweetness

• Anchovies for an extra layer of umami

Step-by-Step Instructions:

1. Prepare Ingredients:

• Ensure that the Kalamata olives are pitted. Drain capers and mince the garlic cloves.

2. Blend Ingredients:

• Combine Kalamata olives, capers, and minced garlic in a food processor. Pulse until the ingredients are finely chopped and well combined.

3. Drizzle Olive Oil:

• While the food processor is running, drizzle in olive oil gradually until the mixture reaches your desired consistency. Depending on your preference, you can make it smoother or keep it slightly chunky.

4. Adjust Seasoning:

• Taste the Olive tapenade and adjust the Seasoning if needed. You can add more garlic, capers, or a splash of lemon juice for brightness.

5. Optional Additions:

• If desired, stir in chopped fresh parsley, lemon zest, sundried tomatoes, or a few anchovies for additional flavors.

6. Serve with Whole Grain Crackers:

• Transfer the Olive Tapenade to a serving bowl. Serve with whole-grain crackers for a wholesome and delicious pairing.

7. Garnish and Enjoy:

• Garnish the Olive Tapenade with additional chopped fresh parsley if desired. Enjoy the savory goodness on each cracker bite.

Note: The nutrition information is an approximate value based on the olives and olive oil used. Actual values may vary depending on specific brands and quantities operated.

CHIA SEED PUDDING WITH COCONUT MILK

Recipe Description: Indulge in a delightful and nutritious treat with Chia Seed Pudding made with Coconut Milk —a luscious combination of chia seeds, creamy coconut milk, and a hint of vanilla extract. This versatile pudding can be enjoyed as a satisfying dessert or a wholesome breakfast. Topped with vibrant berries, it offers a burst of flavors and a pleasing contrast of textures. Embrace the goodness of chia seeds and the tropical richness of coconut milk in every spoonful.

Ingredients:

• Chia seeds

• Coconut milk (full-fat or light)

• Vanilla extract

• Berries for topping (strawberries, blueberries, raspberries, etc.)

Optional Additions:

• Sweetener of choice (maple syrup, honey, agave nectar)

• Shredded coconut for garnish

• Sliced almonds or chopped nuts for crunch

• Mint leaves for a fresh garnish

Step-by-Step Instructions:

1. Mix Chia Seed Pudding Base:

• Combine chia seeds, coconut milk, and vanilla extract in a bowl. Stir well to ensure the chia seeds are evenly distributed.

2. Sweeten to Taste:

• If desired, add a sweetener of your choice (maple syrup, honey, or agave nectar) to the mixture. Adjust the sweetness according to your preference.

3. Refrigerate Overnight:

• Cover the bowl and refrigerate the Chia Seed Pudding mixture overnight or for at least 4-6 hours. This allows the chia seeds to absorb the liquid and create a pudding-like consistency.

4. Stir Before Serving:

• Before serving, give the Chia Seed Pudding a good stir to ensure a uniform texture. If it's too thick, add more coconut milk to reach your desired consistency.

5. Top with Berries:

• Spoon the chia seed pudding into serving glasses or bowls. Top with generous fresh berries such as strawberries, blueberries, or raspberries.

6. Optional Garnishes:

• Garnish with shredded coconut, sliced almonds or chopped nuts, and a few mint leaves for additional flair.

7. Serve and Enjoy:

• Serve the Chia Seed Pudding with Coconut Milk immediately and savor the creamy, nutrient-packed goodness.

Note: The nutrition information is an approximate value based on standard ingredients. Actual values may vary depending on specific brands and quantities used.

PISTACHIO-CRUSTED CHICKEN

Recipe Description: Elevate your chicken dinner with Pistachio-Crusted Chicken—a succulent chicken breast coated in a crunchy pistachios and Dijon mustard layer. This dish boasts a delightful contrast of textures and combines the rich, nutty flavor of pistachios with the zesty kick of Dijon mustard. Serve it as a main course for a special dinner, or impress your guests with this gourmet-inspired dish that's surprisingly easy to make.

Ingredients:

• Chicken breast

• Pistachios, shelled and finely chopped

• Dijon mustard

Optional Additions:

• Fresh herbs (rosemary, thyme) for additional flavor

• Lemon zest for a citrusy kick

• Salt and pepper to taste

Step-by-Step Instructions:

1. Preheat the Oven:

• Preheat your Oven to 400°F (200°C).

2. Prepare Pistachio Coating:

• In a bowl, combine finely chopped pistachios with Dijon mustard. Add fresh herbs, lemon zest, salt, and pepper for additional flavor.

3. Coat Chicken Breast:

• Pat the chicken breast dry with a paper towel. Coat the chicken breast evenly with the pistachio and Dijon mixture, pressing it onto the surface.

4. Sear in a Pan:

• Heat a bit of olive oil over medium-high heat in an oven-safe skillet. Sear the pistachio-crusted chicken breast for 2-3 minutes on each side until golden brown.

5. Transfer to the Oven:

• If using an oven-safe skillet, transfer the entire skillet to the preheated Oven. Alternatively, transfer the seared chicken breast to a baking dish.

6. Bake Until Cooked Through:

• Bake the pistachio-crusted chicken in the Oven for approximately 15-20 minutes or until the internal temperature reaches 165°F (74°C) and the crust is golden and crispy.

7. Rest Before Slicing:

• Allow the chicken to rest for a few minutes before slicing. This helps to retain the juices and ensures a moist chicken breast.

8. Serve and Enjoy:

• Slice the Pistachio-Crusted Chicken and serve it hot. Pair it with your favorite side dishes for a complete and satisfying meal.

Optional Serving Suggestions:

• Serve over a bed of fresh greens or alongside roasted vegetables.

• Drizzle with a balsamic glaze for added sweetness and acidity.

Note: The nutrition information is an approximate value based on standard ingredients. Actual values may vary depending on specific brands and quantities used.

GUACAMOLE WITH VEGGIE STICKS

Recipe Description: Indulge in the vibrant flavors of Guacamole with Veggie Sticks—a refreshing and nutritious snack that brings together the creamy richness of Avocado, the tangy burst of tomatoes and lime, and the crispness of assorted veggies. This crowd-pleasing guacamole is a delicious dip and a wholesome choice for a light and satisfying snack. Pair it with an array of colorful veggie sticks for a delightful combination of textures and tastes.

Ingredients:

• Avocado, ripe

• Tomatoes, diced

• Onion, finely chopped

• Lime, juiced

• Assorted veggies for dipping (carrot sticks, cucumber slices, bell pepper strips, etc.)

Optional Additions:

• Garlic, minced for extra flavor

• Jalapeño, finely chopped, for heat

• Fresh cilantro, chopped for a burst of freshness

• Salt and pepper to taste

Step-by-Step Instructions:

1. Prepare the Guacamole Base:

• Scoop out the ripe Avocado into a bowl. Mash it with a fork until you achieve your desired level of creaminess.

2. Add Tomatoes and Onion:

• Add diced tomatoes and finely chopped onion to the mashed Avocado. Mix well to combine.

3. Squeeze Lime Juice:

• Squeeze the juice of a lime into the guacamole mixture. Lime adds a zesty kick and helps prevent the Avocado from browning.

4. Optional Additions:

• If desired, add minced garlic, finely chopped jalapeño for heat, and fresh cilantro for an extra burst of freshness. Season with salt and pepper to taste.

5. Mix Thoroughly:

• Mix all the ingredients thoroughly to ensure an even distribution of flavors.

6. Prepare Veggie Sticks:

• Wash and cut an assortment of veggies into sticks or slices. Carrot sticks, cucumber slices, and bell pepper strips work well.

7. Serve and Enjoy:

• Arrange the Guacamole with Veggie Sticks on a serving platter. Dive into this fresh and flavorful snack with the colorful assortment of veggie dippers.

Optional Serving Tips:

• Consider adding a sprinkle of crumbled feta or cotija cheese on top for extra richness.

• Serve with whole grain pita wedges or tortilla chips for variety.

Note: The nutrition information is an approximate value based on standard ingredients. Actual values may vary depending on specific brands and quantities used.

COTTAGE CHEESE AND PINEAPPLE BOWL

Recipe Description: Transport yourself to a tropical paradise with the Cottage Cheese and Pineapple Bowl—a simple yet satisfying combination of creamy cottage cheese, sweet and juicy pineapple chunks, and the crunch of sliced almonds. Packed with protein and vitamins, this refreshing bowl makes for a delightful breakfast, snack, or even a light dessert. Enjoy the balance of textures and flavors in every spoonful of this tropical-inspired treat.

Ingredients:

• Cottage cheese

• Fresh pineapple chunks

• Sliced almonds

Optional Additions:

• Honey or maple syrup for sweetness

• Mint leaves for garnish

• Coconut flakes for a tropical touch

Step-by-Step Instructions:

1. Prepare Cottage Cheese Base:

• Scoop a portion of cottage cheese into a bowl. The amount can be adjusted based on your preference.

2. Add Fresh Pineapple Chunks:

• Add a generous amount of fresh pineapple chunks to the cottage cheese. Ensure the pineapple is ripe for optimal sweetness.

3. Sprinkle with Sliced Almonds:

• Sprinkle sliced almonds over the cottage cheese and pineapple. The almonds add a delightful crunch and nutty flavor.

4. Optional Sweetener:

• If desired, drizzle a small amount of honey or maple syrup over the Cottage Cheese and Pineapple Bowl for extra sweetness. Adjust to your liking.

5. Garnish with Mint Leaves:

• Garnish the bowl with fresh mint leaves for a burst of freshness. This step is optional but enhances the overall presentation.

6. Optional Coconut Flakes:

• For a tropical touch, consider sprinkling coconut flakes over the bowl. Coconut adds a hint of sweetness and complements the pineapple flavor.

7. Mix and Enjoy:

• Gently mix the ingredients in the bowl to combine the flavors. Dive into this tropical delight with a spoon and savor the creamy, fruity, and nutty goodness.

Optional Serving Tips:

• Serve the Cottage Cheese and Pineapple Bowl chilled for

a refreshing experience.

• For variety, experiment with other nuts, such as chopped walnuts or pecans.

Note: The nutrition information is an approximate value based on standard ingredients. Actual values may vary depending on specific brands and quantities used.

SESAME GINGER DRESSING

Recipe Description: Elevate your salads, stir-fries, and more with the Sesame Ginger Dressing—a harmonious blend of rich sesame oil, savory soy sauce, zesty ginger, aromatic garlic, and tangy rice vinegar. This versatile dressing adds an explosion of flavors to your dishes, providing a perfect balance of sweetness, saltiness, and umami. Enjoy the culinary magic as this dressing enhances the taste of your favorite meals.

Ingredients:

- Sesame oil

- Soy sauce (low-sodium for a lighter option)

- Fresh ginger, grated

- Garlic, minced

- Rice vinegar

Optional Additions:

- Honey or maple syrup for sweetness

- Sesame seeds for texture

- Green onions, finely chopped, for freshness

- Red pepper flakes for heat

Step-by-Step Instructions:

1. Assemble Ingredients:

• Gather sesame oil, soy sauce, freshly grated ginger, minced garlic, and rice vinegar.

2. Mix Sesame Oil and Soy Sauce:

• In a bowl, combine sesame oil and soy sauce. The ratio can be adjusted to achieve the desired balance of flavors.

3. Add Grated Ginger:

• Grate fresh ginger and add it to the sesame oil and soy sauce mixture. The ginger adds a zesty and aromatic kick.

4. Incorporate Minced Garlic:

• Mince garlic cloves finely and add them to the mixture. Garlic contributes a savory depth to the dressing.

5. Splash of Rice Vinegar:

• Add rice vinegar to the bowl. The vinegar provides a tangy element that enhances the overall flavor profile.

6. Optional Sweetener:

• Add a small amount of honey or maple syrup to the dressing for sweetness if desired. Adjust according to your taste preferences.

7. Optional Texture and Heat:

• For added texture, consider tossing in sesame seeds. Add red pepper flakes to the dressing if you enjoy a bit of heat.

8. Whisk or Shake:

• Whisk the ingredients together thoroughly, place them in a jar with a tight-fitting lid, and shake until well combined.

9. Taste and Adjust:

• Taste the Sesame Ginger Dressing and adjust the flavors by adding more soy sauce, ginger, or sweetener if necessary.

10. Store and Enjoy:

• Store the dressing in a sealed container in the Refrigerator. Shake or whisk before each use. Drizzle over salads, use as a marinade, or enhance stir-fries with this flavorful elixir.

Note: The nutrition information is an approximate value based on standard ingredients. Actual values may vary depending on specific brands and quantities used.

CHAPTER SEVEN

Hydration Recipes

Green Tea and Citrus Infusion

Recipe Description: Quench your thirst with the Green Tea and Citrus Infusion—a revitalizing beverage that combines the antioxidant-rich goodness of green tea with the zesty brightness of orange and lime slices. This refreshing infusion hydrates and provides a burst of flavor and invigorating energy. Whether enjoyed hot or chilled, this delightful beverage is perfect for moments of relaxation or as a pick-me-up throughout the day.

Ingredients:

• Green tea bags

• Water

• Orange slices

• Lime slices

Optional Additions:

• Mint leaves for freshness

• Honey or agave syrup for sweetness

• Ice cubes for a chilled version

Step-by-Step Instructions:

1. Boil Water:

• Bring Water to a boil. The amount of Water can be adjusted based on the number of servings desired.

2. Steep Green Tea Bags:

• Place green tea bags in a teapot or heatproof container. Pour the boiling water over the tea bags and let them steep for 2-3 minutes. Adjust steeping time based on your preference for tea strength.

3. Add Citrus Slices:

• While the tea is still warm, add slices of fresh orange and lime to the pot. The warmth will help release the citrus flavors.

4. Optional Mint Leaves:

• For an extra touch of freshness, add mint leaves to the pot. Crush the leaves slightly to release their aroma.

5. Sweeten if Desired:

• If you prefer a sweeter infusion, add honey or agave syrup to the warm tea and stir until dissolved. Adjust sweetness to taste.

6. Strain and Serve:

• After the infusion has steeped to your liking, strain the tea to remove the tea bags, citrus slices, and mint leaves.

7. Chilled Version:

• If you prefer a chilled version, allow the tea to cool to room temperature, then refrigerate. Serve over ice cubes for a refreshing iced tea.

8. Garnish and Enjoy:

• Garnish individual cups with additional citrus slices or mint leaves. Serve the Green Tea and Citrus Infusion and enjoy the revitalizing blend of flavors.

Note: The nutrition information is an approximate value based on standard ingredients. Actual values may vary depending on specific brands and quantities used.

LEMON GINGER DETOX WATER

Recipe Description: Revitalize your hydration routine with Lemon Ginger Detox Water—a simple yet powerful elixir that combines lemon's cleansing properties with ginger's soothing warmth. This refreshing drink provides a burst of flavor, supports digestion, and helps flush out toxins. Whether you're looking for a daily detox or a flavorful way to increase your water intake, this infused Water is a hydrating choice that's easy to make and enjoyable.

Ingredients:

• Water

• Lemon slices

• Ginger slices

Optional Additions:

• Fresh mint leaves for a hint of freshness

• Cucumber slices for added hydration

• Honey or agave syrup for a touch of sweetness

Step-by-Step Instructions:

1. Prepare Water:

• Fill a pitcher or water bottle with the desired amount of

Water. Use filtered or still Water for the best taste.

2. Add Lemon Slices:

• Slice a fresh lemon, and add the lemon slices to the Water. Adjust the quantity based on your preference for lemon flavor.

3. Add Ginger Slices:

• Peel and slice fresh ginger into thin rounds. Add the ginger slices to the Water. Start with a small amount and adjust to your taste preferences.

4. Optional Mint Leaves:

• Add a few fresh mint leaves to the Water for an extra burst of freshness. Crush them slightly to release their aroma.

5. Optional Cucumber Slices:

• Enhance the hydration by adding cucumber slices to the mix. Cucumber adds a subtle and refreshing taste.

6. Optional Sweetener:

• If you prefer a sweeter flavor, consider adding a small amount of honey or agave syrup to the detox water. Stir well to dissolve.

7. Chill and Infuse:

• Place the pitcher or water bottle in the Refrigerator and let the Lemon Ginger Detox Water chill for at least a couple of hours or overnight. This allows the flavors to infuse into the Water.

8. Serve and Enjoy:

• Pour the chilled detox water into glasses. If desired, add ice cubes for an extra refreshing touch. Sip and enjoy the hydrating and cleansing benefits.

Note: The nutrition information is an approximate value based on standard ingredients. Actual values may vary depending on specific brands and quantities used.

CUCUMBER LEMONADE

Recipe Description: Beat the heat with a glass of Cucumber Lemonade—a cooling and revitalizing beverage that combines the crispness of Cucumber with the zesty tang of lemon. Sweetened with agave syrup, this homemade lemonade is a delightful and healthier alternative to store-bought options. Cucumber Lemonade is easy to make and sure to become a favorite in your repertoire, perfect for hot summer days or any time you crave a refreshing drink.

Ingredients:

• Cucumber peeled and sliced

• Lemon juice (freshly squeezed)

• Agave syrup (adjust to taste)

• Water

• Ice cubes for serving

Optional Additions:

• Mint leaves for extra freshness

• Lemon slices for garnish

• Sparkling Water for a fizzy variation

Step-by-Step Instructions:

1. Prepare Cucumber:

• Peel and slice the Cucumber into thin rounds. The cucumber slices will be used to infuse the lemonade with a refreshing taste.

2. Squeeze Lemon Juice:

• Extract fresh lemon juice by squeezing lemons. Adjust the quantity based on your preference for tartness.

3. Mix Cucumber, Lemon Juice, and Agave Syrup:

• Combine the cucumber slices, freshly squeezed lemon juice, and agave syrup in a pitcher. Start with a small amount of agave syrup and adjust to your desired level of sweetness.

4. Muddle Mint Leaves (Optional):

• For an extra burst of freshness, muddle a few mint leaves and add them to the pitcher. This step is optional but adds a delightful herbal note.

5. Add Water:

• Pour Water into the pitcher and stir well to combine all the ingredients. Adjust the water quantity based on your preferred concentration.

6. Chill in the Refrigerator:

• Place the pitcher in the Refrigerator and let the Cucumber Lemonade chill for at least 1-2 hours. This allows the flavors to meld and the drink to become thoroughly chilled.

7. Serve Over Ice:

• When ready to serve, fill glasses with ice cubes and pour the chilled Cucumber Lemonade over the ice.

8. Garnish and Enjoy:

• Garnish each glass with a slice of lemon or a cucumber wheel. Stir and enjoy this cool and revitalizing summer drink.

Note: The nutrition information is an approximate value based on standard ingredients. Actual values may vary depending on specific brands and quantities used.

SPARKLING WATER WITH LEMON AND BERRIES

Recipe Description: Elevate your hydration experience with Sparkling Water with Lemon and Berries—a bubbly and flavorful drink that combines the effervescence of sparkling Water with the citrusy kick of lemon slices and the sweetness of mixed berries. This refreshing beverage is a delightful alternative to sugary sodas and a visually appealing and hydrating option for any occasion. Enjoy the fizzy sensation and the burst of natural flavors in every sip.

Ingredients:

• Sparkling Water

• Lemon slices

• Mixed berries (strawberries, blueberries, raspberries, etc.)

Optional Additions:

• Mint leaves for a touch of freshness

• Honey or agave syrup for sweetness

• Ice cubes for extra chill

Step-by-Step Instructions:

1. Prepare Ingredients:

• Wash and slice fresh lemon into rounds. Rinse the mixed berries and set them aside.

2. Fill Glasses with Sparkling Water:

• Fill individual glasses with sparkling Water. Adjust the quantity based on the number of servings desired.

3. Squeeze Lemon Juice:

• Squeeze a bit of lemon juice into each glass to add a citrusy kick. Adjust the amount to your taste preference.

4. Add Lemon Slices and Berries:

• Drop lemon slices into the glasses for visual appeal and an extra burst of lemon flavor. Add a handful of mixed berries to each glass.

5. Optional Sweetener:

• Add a small amount of honey or agave syrup if you prefer a sweeter drink. Stir well to dissolve the sweetener.

6. Add Mint Leaves (Optional):

• Add a few mint leaves to each glass for a touch of freshness. Crush them slightly to release their aroma.

7. Optional Ice Cubes:

• If you enjoy extra chill, add ice cubes to the glasses. The ice enhances the refreshing quality of the drink.

8. Stir Gently:

• Give the ingredients a gentle stir to distribute the flavors and ensure an even mix of berries and lemon throughout the sparkling Water.

9. Serve and Enjoy:

• Present the Sparkling Water with Lemon and Berries glasses to your guests, or enjoy them yourself. Sip and savor the effervescence and fruity goodness.

Note: The nutrition information is an approximate value based on standard ingredients. Actual values may vary depending on specific brands and quantities used.

CONCLUSION

In conclusion, the intricate dance between diet and stroke prevention or recovery underscores the pivotal role that our food choices play in shaping the trajectory of our health. The journey through the realms of a stroke-conscious diet reveals a profound connection between the foods we consume and the well-being of our cardiovascular system, particularly the delicate balance required for optimal brain function.

A stroke diet, far from being a restrictive set of rules, emerges as a roadmap to a healthier and more resilient life. It is a testament to the power of proactive, mindful choices that not only mitigate the risk of stroke but also support recovery for those who have experienced this life-altering event. From the vibrant colors of antioxidant-rich fruits and vegetables to the heart-healthy embrace of omega-3 fatty acids found in fish, the strokes of our culinary palette can indeed paint a picture of sustained well-being.

Portion control, a reduction in sodium intake, and the thoughtful exclusion of processed sugars are not merely guidelines; they are keystones in the construction of a fortress against stroke. A diet that values the quality of nutrients over the quantity of calories becomes a shield, guarding against the insidious risk factors that lurk within our modern lifestyles.

Yet, the stroke diet is not a solitary hero in this narrative. It harmoniously resonates with the rhythm of a broader lifestyle melody. Regular physical activity, maintaining a healthy weight, and effective stress management compose the symphony of a holistic approach to cardiovascular health. Together, these components create a resilient tapestry woven with threads of care and commitment to one's well-being.

As we traverse the landscape of stroke awareness and dietary mindfulness, let us recognize that our choices today echo into the vitality of our tomorrows. Consulting healthcare professionals for personalized guidance becomes a compass, guiding us through the unique contours of our health landscapes.

In embracing the principles of a stroke-conscious diet, we embark on a journey of self-care and empowerment, not solely about avoiding the pitfalls of illness but about nurturing the fullness of life. With each mindful bite and every heart-healthy meal, we contribute to the canvas of our own longevity, painting strokes that echo the promise of a healthier tomorrow.

www.ingramcontent.com/pod-product-compliance
Lightning Source LLC
Chambersburg PA
CBHW070941250726
48663CB00001B/18